Prais

T

BAD FOOD BIBLE

"*The Bad Food Bible* changed the way I eat and look at food (sounds hyperbolic but I'm serious, the book is amazing)."
— Alex Beggs, *Bon Appetit*

"This excellent title from Carroll explains that practically no food or drink is as bad as certain 'studies show' data would have us believe . . . VERDICT: An excellent choice for every reader and all collections." — *Library Journal*, starred review

"*The Bad Food Bible* knocks down a number of nutrition myths . . . [Carroll] closes the book with nine common-sense rules for healthy eating." — *Wall Street Journal*

"In this informative, accessible book, Carroll, a doctor and healthcare expert, sifts through the research, advice, and straight-up hype surrounding diets to reveal that some of the foods we view as off-limits aren't as awful as we think . . . The book has plenty of sensible tips for maintaining a healthy diet . . . Here's to a delicious new year!" — *BookPage*

"The cacophony of dietary doctrine has reached a fever pitch . . . Carroll uses historical examples and rarely published scientific evidence to help us see through the current pandemonium. His commonsense approach lays the groundwork for a healthy relationship with 'sinful' foods." — *iBooks*

"*The Bad Food Bible* is a breath of fresh air in a media environment saturated with eating dos and don'ts. For anyone confused by single-study headlines or looking to make sense of how to eat healthy with a world of so many options, Aaron Carroll's advice will certainly deliver."
— Sarah Kliff, senior policy correspondent, Vox.com

"Eat, drink, and relax, already. As Aaron Carroll shows in *The Bad Food Bible*, when it comes to nutritional health, much of what we've been told to worry about is either hyped or hogwash." — Michael Moss, best-selling author of *Salt Sugar Fat*

"Aaron Carroll's brilliant advice has changed my health and my life. Forget about all the fads: here's the real truth about food and the role it plays in our lives."
— John Green, best-selling author of *The Fault in Our Stars*

"A satisfying book that challenges the very notion of food morality and frees us up for some seriously delicious, sinful eating."
— Nina Teicholz, best-selling author of *The Big Fat Surprise*

"In *The Bad Food Bible*, Aaron Carroll turns down the food fear sirens to zero, and responsibly explains what science actually says about the food we eat. Instead of demonizing prosciutto or wine, Carroll reminds us that the odd indulgence isn't going to kill anyone, but a lifetime of poor nutrition might — sane and welcome advice in a time of great nutrition confusion."
— Julia Belluz, senior health correspondent, Vox.com

The

BAD FOOD
BIBLE

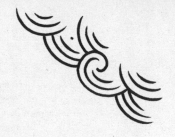

The
BAD FOOD
BIBLE

WHY YOU CAN
(AND MAYBE SHOULD)
EAT EVERYTHING YOU
THOUGHT YOU COULDN'T

AARON CARROLL, MD

MARINER BOOKS
HOUGHTON MIFFLIN HARCOURT
BOSTON   NEW YORK

First Mariner Books edition 2019
Copyright © 2017 by Aaron Carroll
Foreword copyright © 2017 by Nina Teicholz
Illustrations © Jim Tierney

For information about permission to reproduce selections from this book,
write to trade.permissions@hmhco.com or to Permissions, Houghton Mifflin Harcourt
Publishing Company, 3 Park Avenue, 19th Floor, New York, New York 10016.

hmhco.com

Library of Congress Cataloging-in-Publication Data
Names: Carroll, Aaron E., author.
Title: The bad food bible : why you can (and maybe should)
eat everything you thought you couldn't / Aaron Carroll, M.D.
Description: Boston : Houghton Mifflin Harcourt, 2017. |
Includes bibliographical references and index.
Identifiers: LCCN 2017044244 (print) | LCCN 2017047377 (ebook) |
ISBN 9780544952577 (ebook) | ISBN 9780544952560 (paper over board) |
ISBN 9781328505774 (pbk.)
Subjects: LCSH: Nutrition--Popular works. | BISAC: MEDICAL / Nutrition. |
COOKING / Health & Healing / General.
Classification: LCC QP141 (ebook) | LCC QP141 .C315 2017 (print) |
DDC 613.2/5—dc23
LC record available at https://lccn.loc.gov/2017044244

Book design by Brian Moore

Printed in the United States of America
DOC 10 9 8 7 6 5 4 3 2 1

Portions of this book appeared, in different form, in the *New York Times*.

For Aimee,
because she doesn't get nearly enough credit.
She also makes everything in my life better — even what I eat.

CONTENTS

FOREWORD

WE live in hard times for people who simply want to eat — normally, that is, in a way that would be recognizable to our ancestors, aiming for no more than a tasty meal, eaten to satisfaction, with a feeling of pleasure. Now, instead, we sit down to dinner in trepidation, our heads swirling with a chorus of wasps whispering, *Eat only good foods; beware the bad.* This moral freight has weighed so heavily on our food choices that one would expect insurrection to be just around the corner. And, indeed, here it is: *The Bad Food Bible,* a satisfying book that challenges the very notion of food morality and frees us up for some seriously delicious, sinful eating.

Dr. Aaron Carroll is no knee-jerk heretic. A thoughtful professor of pediatrics who came to the field of nutrition on a simple quest to learn how better to advise his patients, as well as improve his own diet, he found himself mired in the inevitable, dizzying array of experts with "radically different opinions" about diet, doused in heavy, judgmental language. We don't need an opinion poll to know that Americans are weary of feeling guilty and confused about their food choices. Carroll feels the same, and in his efforts to drill down to some nutritional terra firma, he's taken a refreshingly rigorous scientific approach.

That is to say, Carroll earns his contrarian views the hard

way. Not only does he dig into a great deal of scientific literature, but, more important, he also weighs and prioritizes it. This is a far more rare and valiant feat than you might imagine.

One of the biggest problems in nutrition over the past fifty years has been how all data — the good and bad, the weak and strong, alike — have been stirred into one big, undifferentiated pot. Evidence from so-called observational studies, which can only show associations, has been given equal footing with a more rigorous kind of data, from randomized controlled trials. As Carroll explains, only the latter can demonstrate cause and effect, and only the latter can justifiably be used for population-wide nutrition recommendations. Yet health experts have strayed far from this narrow path.

Like most things, this homogenization of data started off with good intentions. Given the complexities of trying to figure out how a lifetime of dietary and lifestyle habits drive disease or death decades later, nutrition science has long been notoriously difficult. It began in the 1950s. Although the data from this period were poor, the rising tide of cardiovascular deaths over previous decades pressured experts into saying *something* about a disease-proof diet. So they did, based on premature findings — with the result being that much of the early advice was simply wrong.

As Carroll writes, "Scientists and doctors are often guilty of acting without sufficient evidence — of making recommendations without having sufficient facts. Most of the time, they're trying to do the right thing. But in some cases, their efforts can have the opposite effect."

That, he says, is the "dirty little secret of medical science."

Carroll discusses the original, big mistakes — on butter, meat, eggs, and salt — in the opening chapters of this book. These long-standing, seemingly rock-solid pillars of conventional dietary wisdom have toppled, either partially or completely, in recent years. As of 2015, American health authorities have dropped their caps on dietary cholesterol — the reason we avoided eggs and shellfish for decades. And over the past five years, teams of researchers all over the world have challenged long-held beliefs about whether "lower is better" regarding salt and whether our avoidance of meat and butter is based on solid evidence. The science on all these points, it turns out, is far from settled.

With fascinating detail, Carroll also tackles more recent disputes over genetically modified organisms (GMOs), organic foods, diet soda, gluten, alcohol, and more. These are all topics on which nutrition science has made substantial advancements, yet old habits remain, with many health experts still sifting hard data indiscriminatingly into soft. Carroll is a warm and engaging guide, with funny stories to share about his own eating habits and those of his family, but when it comes to the science, he takes no prisoners. On each of these contested topics, he weighs the evidence carefully and follows the data, even when they lead to conclusions that are inconvenient or unpopular.

On diet soda, for instance, he writes, "I don't think that letting my children drink diet soda once in a while makes me a monster, but apparently some people do." What's more, people seem "to object to the *diet* even more than to the *soda*." Yet we know more about the dangers of sugar than artificial sweeteners, he notes, and the occasional diet soda isn't going to kill anyone.

This is just one example of the fearmongering that Carroll chides. This demonization of certain foods is fanned by advocacy groups and experts alike, and leaves ordinary people susceptible to terrible advice about their diets. Food phobias paralyze people, to the point where they literally don't know which supermarket aisle to walk down. This uncertainty turns out to be the perfect culture in which ideology, industry tricks, and commonplace charlatanism flourish, leading to diets of all kinds based less on basic nutrition than on aspirations, passion, and, yes, even the freedom from sin.

Maybe it's ironic that Carroll calls his book a food *bible* when the only preaching he's doing is good old-fashioned science, but his ultimate point is that we should back away from faith-based eating and just eat *real* food — you know, the kind that our ancestors would have recognized. Plus, perhaps, the occasional diet soda, if you want. No guilt.

"Eating is one of the great joys of life. Don't let people use misinformation or bad science to deprive you of the pleasure of good food," Carroll writes. Amen to that.

NINA TEICHOLZ

Nina Teicholz is an investigative journalist and author of the international and *New York Times* bestseller, *The Big Fat Surprise*. The *Economist* named it a top science book of 2014, and it was also named a 2014 Best Book by the *Wall Street Journal, Forbes, Mother Jones,* and *Library Journal*. Before taking a deep dive into researching nutrition science, Teicholz was a reporter for NPR and also contributed to many publications, including the *Wall Street Journal*, the *New York Times,* the *Washington Post, The New Yorker,* and the *Economist*. She attended Yale and Stanford, where she studied biology and majored in American studies. She has a master's degree from Oxford University and served as associate director of the Center on Globalization and Sustainable Development at Columbia University. She lives in New York City.

INTRODUCTION

R ECENTLY, an old friend of mine was in town for a visit. He loves food, as do my wife and I, so we took him out to a nice restaurant here in Indiana. When it came time to order our entrées, I found myself in an all-too-common predicament: Should I order the "healthy" option or the one that sounded the tastiest?

Luckily, I've become somewhat of an expert on this type of dilemma, and so I chose the tenderloin. It proved to be one of the best pieces of meat I've ever eaten. My wife and our friend ordered dishes they thought were healthier. They didn't seem to enjoy their meals as much as I did, but they could console themselves with the knowledge that they had made the "right" choice in the long run.

Had they? It depends on whom you ask.

Today, self-professed experts of all stripes — from doctors to dieticians, weight-loss gurus to personal trainers, bloggers to YouTubers, and everyone in between — seem to have radically different opinions about what we should be eating, and why. All of these viewpoints, well-intentioned though they may be, buffet us with wave after wave of dietary advice that promises to make us thinner, cure us of disease (or prevent it entirely), and ultimately extend our lives. *We should eat like cavemen did. We should avoid gluten completely. We should eat only organic. Or vegetarian. Or vegan.* These different waves of advice push us in one direction, then another. More often than not, we end up right where we started, but with thinner wallets and thicker waistlines.

If you have a hard time keeping all of these recommendations straight, or choosing between them, you're not alone. I'm a physician and researcher who has a particular interest in analyzing dietary health research, and even I find my head spinning when I think about the number of different perspectives on something as seemingly simple as the benefits of brown rice or the dangers of red meat. This is one of the reasons I decided to focus much of my writing on dietary health. I wanted to be able to advise my patients about what healthy eating looks like — and I also wanted to practice it myself.

These conflicting opinions about food have one thing in common: the belief that some foods will kill you — or, at the very least, that those foods are the reason you're not at the weight you'd like to be. This is an attitude about food that, ironically, has its roots in an earlier and opposite idea: that some foods can keep us from dying. Indeed, some of the earliest "expert" advice about food was predicated on the notion that some foods can save us.

The first nutritional guidelines endorsed by the U.S. Department of Agriculture, which appeared in 1894, were a product of the times. In the late nineteenth century, people in the United States were eating more calories and consuming more meat and fish than people in most other countries in the world. Even so, many Americans were malnourished. Rickets, beriberi, and scurvy — conditions that are caused by nutritional deficiencies — were much more common then than they are today. As a result, experts' dietary recommendations focused on eating a variety of foods in a balanced way to overcome those deficits.

At that time, however, the links between specific components of foods and health problems were vague. That began to change in the twentieth century, when scientists started figuring out how to identify vitamins and minerals in the lab. They better understood how individual nutrients, vitamins, and minerals were related to health and well-being. These breakthroughs led governments around the world to implement policies and guidelines that encouraged people to eat foods rich in, or fortified with, components such as vitamins D, B, and C. These efforts worked. Rickets, beriberi, and scurvy are nearly unheard-of in the developed world.

Those early successes gave many people the impression that some foods have medicinal properties. But what's true for vitamin deficiencies isn't necessarily true for other illnesses. Cutting certain kinds of food out of your diet altogether isn't guaranteed to cure a disease; sometimes, in fact, it can actually harm you.

Today, the number one killer in much of the Western world is heart disease. We've struggled to come up with nutritional guidelines that can put a dent in the problem. By the 1970s, for example, some scientists came to believe that we were eating too much of some nutrients, especially fats. The nutritional guidelines began to advise us to avoid fats and the meats that accompany them. We were told that those things would kill us.

It seemed like sensible advice at the time. But now, several decades after those guidelines were developed, it looks like they may have made things worse. When people cut fats and meat out of their diets, they must eat something else. For diners in the late twentieth century, this meant turning to grains and other carbohydrates. The results weren't pretty. Obesity rates shot through the roof, as did the incidence of diabetes and heart disease.

As it turns out, meat and fats were never really the danger researchers and health care professionals made them out to be — at least not to the extent that many experts claimed. Nor was cholesterol. But even as we've begun to appreciate these facts, we have found other foods to blame for our problems. Today, we focus on new "dangers," including gluten, genetically modified organisms (GMOs), and artificial sweeteners. None of these things are as dangerous as you might think, either—but that hasn't stopped medical experts and laypeople alike from demonizing them.

These reactions and counter-reactions point to an uncomfortable truth about the field of dietary health. Scientists and doctors are often guilty of acting without sufficient evidence —of making recommendations without having sufficient facts. Most of the time, they're trying to do the right thing. But in some cases, their efforts can have the opposite effect.

THE DIRTY LITTLE SECRET OF MEDICAL SCIENCE

Babies spit up. A lot. When this spitting up becomes a problem —when it causes them pain or interferes with weight gain— their parents often bring them to the doctor. When it gets really bad, pediatricians like me give it a fancy name: gastroesophageal reflux disease, or GERD.

Because doctors like to fix problems, pediatricians are likely to recommend any number of interventions to treat GERD in infants. Many of these recommendations are nutritional. For instance, we might advise parents to thicken their babies' feeds or change the formula they're using. If these fixes don't work, we might recommend putting their babies in an infant seat, giving them a pacifier, or having them sleep on a wedge.

None of these treatments actually work, but the last one may be the least effective of all. A wedge is a foam incline, about two feet long, that is sloped to reach a height of about one foot on one end. When I was a resident, the hospital in which I was training would create wedges for patients upon request. They made a ton of them and charged about $150 apiece. Insurance didn't cover the wedges, but many parents — thinking that their babies' health was at stake — somehow came up with the cash.

I had a hard time believing the wedges were worth the cost, so I set out to find evidence in the medical literature to support their use. I couldn't find any. When I challenged doctors about this, I would get all kinds of responses. *Patients who were put on wedges got better. Doctors and others they knew swore by them. Parents didn't mind the wedges, and they were easy to use. What's the harm?*

My colleagues who defended prescribing wedges weren't entirely wrong when they said that babies who were put on them got better. That's because babies with GERD are almost always not sick.

Infants vomit because they have an all-liquid diet. They also have an immature esophageal sphincter, which doesn't quite close off the stomach from the esophagus, therefore allowing stomach acid to travel the wrong way through their digestive tract. They eat every few hours, and they have a small stomach. Countless infants have symptoms of gastroesophageal reflux. About 95% of infants who have GERD get better on their own. Therefore, anything we do, whether it's thickening their feeds, changing their formula, or giving them a wedge, makes no difference at all. The wedge appears to work because as time passes, the infants start sitting up and then walking, and they also start eating solid food.

The *appearance* of success was enough to convince many doctors that wedges were successful. Because the babies they put on wedges got better, they assumed that wedges worked. They weren't ignoring the evidence; it just wasn't good evidence.

These doctors were, however, ignoring many of the downsides to wedges. Parents often hated them. They were a pain to carry around, and many moms and dads feared letting their infants even nap without them. This meant they had to purchase additional wedges for other places where their babies might spend a lot of time, such as day care or grandparents' houses. Some babies didn't like sleeping on them and were fussier at night. More often than not, it seemed, wedges were causing parents and infants to suffer while making the families poorer — all without actually doing any good.

I decided I had to set the record straight. So in my free time (and there wasn't much of it back when I was a resident), I deepened my search, scouring the medical literature even more thoroughly to make sure I hadn't missed anything. I reviewed more than 2,500 studies and identified 35 that might discuss the use of these nonpharmacologic and nonsurgical therapies in the treatment of infant GERD.

Eventually, ten randomized controlled trials* met the criteria I was looking for. Those ten trials proved that none of the therapies I mentioned above seemed to work. The paper based on this work was my first official publication, and the first step on the road to my becoming a medical researcher.

What surprised me wasn't that my paper got published, but that it was so widely read. It is still one of my most cited pieces. This is not because it broke new ground, but because it gathered and explained the research behind a common problem in a systematic and usable way — something that, alas, health experts do not do nearly enough.

This is the dirty little secret of medical science: Much of what we do, as doctors, is a "best guess." Very few of the recommendations we make are scientifically proven or based on a medical consensus that we are absolutely sure is true. Even more dis-

---

* I promise I will explain what these are in just a little bit. Keep reading.

turbingly, when good evidence does exist, too often we ignore it. The wedge paper offered me my first glimpse of this sad fact, and as the years passed, I became increasingly dismayed by it — and more and more determined to bring it to light.

The root of the problem is this: all research is not created equal. Everyone knows that on some level. How many times have you tuned in to the news to hear about some new miracle advance, only to see years later that it didn't pan out? How many vitamins have been announced as the "key" to living longer, to building more muscle, or to losing weight? Years later, however, they go out of vogue, and we latch onto the next shiny object.

I became so frustrated with these obstacles to good decision making about human health that I decided my time would be better spent trying to get physicians and the health care system to do the right, proven thing than trying to get patients to do what doctors might "think" is right. This is how, eventually, I ended up at Indiana University School of Medicine, working as a health services researcher and directing the school's Center for Health Policy and Professionalism Research.

In the past few years, I've also had the good fortune to write a column for the *New York Times* focusing on data, evidence, and research, and explaining to readers how those things relate to health and health policy. Many of my columns have been about nutrition; in fact, those columns have been among my most popular. My growing body of work in this area — as well as my realization that food is perhaps the best entrée into the important but often dry subject of health research — led to this book.

People have a real hunger for scientific evidence about dietary health, and I take joy in feeding it to them. I relish breaking down complex research and describing what science actually says about what we should eat. Often this involves killing a sacred cow or two, but the upside is that by debunking bad claims about food, I often clear the way for good news.

I have good news and bad news for you at the outset of this book. The bad news is that you are likely worrying too much about some of the foods you eat and feeling too positive about others. The good news is that there's a solution.

In this book, I'm going to teach you how to think about nutrition better and how not to worry so much about many of the things you've been told about food — especially the warnings to stay away from certain ingredients or categories of ingredients because they're "bad for you," full stop.

As with the backlash against fats in the 1970s, when we tell people to cut certain foods out of their diets completely, their health usually suffers. The fact is, practically none of the food you find in a supermarket will kill you unless it's gone bad or you eat way too much of it. Of course, some people are allergic to certain foods, or have medical conditions that require them to limit their intake more than they would have to otherwise. But unless your doctor has told you to avoid specific ingredients for those reasons, the watchword is *moderation,* not abstinence.

If there's one message I want you to take away from this book, it's that you should feel free to enjoy almost any food, even the most "sinful," without worrying that it will negatively impact your health. More important than what you're eating is how you're eating it — especially how often and how much. Anyone who tells you different is likely relying on wrong or incomplete information.

In the pages to come, I'll lay out some rules of thumb for enjoying a healthy relationship with the supposedly most unhealthy foods. But to understand how I've come to these conclusions, you need to know what kind of evidence you should pay attention to, and what kind you can safely disregard.

HOW TO RATE A SCIENTIFIC STUDY

The first thing to remember when you read a new research finding about dietary health is that human beings are really complicated animals. The reasons we eat certain foods — or do anything else, for that matter — are far more complex than they are for most, if not all, other organisms. They're certainly much more complex than they are for isolated cells or cultures in test tubes. Therefore, any study that involves only chemicals or animals in a lab should be taken with a grain of salt. I'm not saying that such research is wrong, per se. I'm just saying that it needs to be replicated and studied in actual people before we can assume it really applies to humans.

This is especially true when it comes to research using animals such as mice or rats. Small-animal research is ubiquitous in the nutrition sciences, despite the fact that it has been shown to be flawed time and time again. Sometimes it's flawed because studies of the ways mice eat just do not translate into accurate conclusions about the ways humans eat. Sometimes it's because such studies use huge amounts of food over short periods of time, which also doesn't necessarily model human behavior. Some mice studies rely on only a few animals, or on animals that are genetically very similar, or they don't use female mice. (When researchers study mice, they want to be able to control as many factors as possible. They also want the mice to be as similar as possible, and they don't want to have to worry about hormonal differences or, even worse, pregnant females. Because of this, it's often easier not to use female mice — a scientific shortcut that also undermines the implications of any such research for humans.)

The bottom line is that you should be suspicious of any dietary advice that's predicated on research involving only chemicals or animals. That's not enough. To make claims about human health, we need human studies.

Even when it comes to human studies, there's a hierarchy of research to consider — a scale of rigor and reliability that tells us to trust some studies more than others, and even discount certain classes of scientific "evidence" altogether.

The lowest form of research is the *anecdote*. That's just a story. For instance: "My great-grandmother ate a tablespoon of Tabasco every morning, and she lived to be nearly a hundred." We hear stories like this all the time. It could be our story or someone else's story, but either way it's no more than one example. Anecdotes, with few exceptions, have no scientific worth whatsoever.

Just above the anecdote in the hierarchy of research is the *case series*. This is a glorified collection of anecdotes, a description of a few examples with no statistical tests to determine whether relationships between factors really exist and how sure of those relationships the researchers might be. Imagine reading a paper describing ten people who ate a tablespoon of Tabasco every day and happened to be very healthy. That would be a case series. It's always been my suspicion that case series were invented by researchers who just wanted to make their anecdotes sound more official. Treat case series with as much disdain as you do individual stories.

The next kind of research — and the first kind that we might take seriously — is the *cross-sectional study*. These studies usually look at a random set of people at a certain point in time to see how one factor might relate to another. Every time you read or hear about a survey talking about how many people do one thing or another, such as eating a tablespoon of Tabasco every day, that's a cross-sectional study. This type of study is great for showing how different people do the same thing — how many men eat meat, for example, or how many young adults are on a certain kind of diet — but not much more.

Next up is the *case-control study*. In this type of research, scientists gather a bunch of people who have a certain condition (*cases*) along with similar people — perhaps those with the same age, sex, and geographic location — who don't have that condition (*controls*). Then the researchers use statistics to see how the people with that condition are different from those without it. Imagine that we gather a bunch of people who have stomach cancer and another bunch of people who don't; ask both groups if, and perhaps how often, they eat a tablespoon of Tabasco; and then analyze the results. This would qualify as a case-control study. Studies like this are better than the ones previously discussed, but they can suffer from what's known as recall bias. When people think about things that occurred in the past, they're more likely to remember those things one way if they're sick and another way if they're not. This kind of bias shows up all the time in health research, including dietary studies. People who have a rare disease are more likely to report having eaten certain things — especially if they've heard that those things are "bad" — than people who are healthy.

An even better type of research is the *cohort study*. This is when a group of people (the cohort) are followed over time in an attempt to discern how certain factors affect them differently — for instance, how certain foods might cause them to gain weight or contract disease. In our Tabasco example, we might keep track of which of them eat a tablespoon of Tabasco every day, wait to see what health patterns emerge among them, and then try to link these patterns to their Tabasco intake. Cohort studies are either retrospective (when researchers gather people and measure stuff that happened to them in the past) or prospective (when they gather people and measure what happens to them over time in the future). For the most part, they're better than case-control studies and less subject to recall bias — but they're still imperfect.

Every one of the studies I've discussed up to this point qualifies as an *observational study*. This class of research can only establish associations, or correlations, between different variables; it cannot prove that one thing causes another. It can tell us, for instance, that people who consume Tabasco are more likely to be overweight, but that doesn't mean that Tabasco necessarily causes weight gain. Another factor could be involved. Perhaps people who eat Tabasco also eat a lot of meat, and that's what makes them heavier.*

Mistaking correlation for causation is one of the most prevalent problems in reporting on health research, including research on dietary health. Way too often, the media latches onto an observational study that has linked some food to some health problem and then reports that the former causes the latter. Observational studies simply cannot prove that.

To prove causation, not simply correlation, we need an *experimental study*. That's when we take a group of people and split them up. Some people get one thing (say, a certain drug or diet), and the others get something else. In an ideal study, researchers also place participants into these groups randomly, so that no one involved in the study has any control over which subjects get which intervention. That way, the researchers can be sure that any differences they see between the groups are caused by the thing they are studying, not by some other factor. Further, the very best studies are controlled by giving a placebo to the group that doesn't receive the thing being studied. In this way, neither the participants nor the people conducting the study know what's going on, and thus cannot inadver-

---

* Not true, by the way.

tently influence the results. This sort of experimental study — the highest form — is called a *randomized controlled trial (RCT)*.

When it comes to determining the impact of diet on human health, RCTs are the gold standard; they are leagues above observational studies. This is because RCTs are pretty much the only kind of studies that can establish causality — that can consistently prove that one thing causes another.

Randomized controlled trials are also exceedingly rare. It's not hard to see why: to conduct one, researchers have to gather many people together, properly enroll them, figure out what to do to them, run the studies while keeping track of everyone for a period of time, measure the results, and then analyze them. I've run a couple of RCTs in my career, and they can cost millions of dollars and be very difficult to conduct.

Because RCTs are so hard to come by, almost everything we "know" about dietary health is based on small, flawed observational studies. The conclusions we can draw from them are limited, and the results are often oversold by researchers and the media. This is the case not only for more recent studies but also for the older research that forms the basis for much of what we currently believe to be true.

Luckily, though good studies are hard to come by, researchers have ways of maximizing their impact. We can do a *systematic review*, gathering good research together and summarizing what it says. Or we can conduct a *meta-analysis*, in which we take the collected research, usually from RCTs, merge the data as best we can, and then analyze it all together as though it were one huge study.

I try to cite meta-analyses and systematic reviews whenever I discuss studies, and I have held myself to that standard in this book as much as possible. Instead of focusing on single studies, I try to talk about a body of research. And where I do cite individual studies, I try to cite RCTs or large cohort studies, and try to place them in the context of the medical literature. I favor studies of humans over rats, and real outcomes (such as heart attacks or deaths) over process measures (such as high blood pressure or cholesterol levels). Process measures are linked to, and perhaps even lead to, the outcomes we really care about, but the information they provide is not as reliable as data on the outcomes themselves and can be flawed.

Throughout this book, I talk about how lesser-quality research has often led us to make bad nutritional decisions. I also point out how good research has been ignored. But because most of the existing research on dietary health is fundamentally limited in terms of its implications for healthy human adults, I debunk many myths about "bad" foods — and, by extension, present a lot of good news about ingredients you love but thought you couldn't have.

THE LIMITS OF NUTRITIONAL SCIENCE

In 2015, a study published in the *Journal of Nutrition* was quickly picked up by the popular media. According to many news reports, the study proved that honey is no healthier than sucrose (i.e., sugar), and that high-fructose corn syrup is no worse.

These announcements shocked people on all sides of the sweetener debate. It had become an article of faith among many people that natural sweeteners like honey are better for you than engineered sweeteners like high-fructose corn syrup, especially if you are concerned about diabetes.

If you looked past these reports and read the scientific study in question, however, you might have noticed something peculiar about the researchers' methods. The study involved only fifty-five people, and they were followed for only *two weeks* as they consumed each of the three sweeteners. The researchers also looked at things like insulin levels, which are lab values that don't translate easily into concepts that people generally understand, such as weight and disease.

The truth is that this was a small, short-lived trial that didn't focus on actual health outcomes. But you wouldn't have known that if you only read the headlines that breathlessly pronounced honey, sugar, and corn syrup of equal health value.

Health research is often misinterpreted, even when it's solid. And this study was perfectly solid. It's among the stronger studies available to us, because it's a randomized controlled trial. But its findings were blown out of proportion by the media, whose reports, in turn, were taken at face value by a scientifically illiterate public.

It's not just reporters and consumers who are to blame for the general lack of understanding about dietary health, however. Nutritional science itself is often fundamentally flawed — and, unfortunately, it shows no sign of improving.

Part of the problem is that clinical trials like this one are often limited in scope. This fact is vividly demonstrated by a 2011 systematic review that identified fifty-three randomized controlled trials looking at the effects of sweeteners on participants' health. That may sound like a lot of research, but only thirteen of the trials lasted for more than a week and involved at least ten (yes, *ten*) participants. Ten of those thirteen trials scored next to last on a standard scale that measures the quality of experimental trials.* None of the trials adequately concealed

---

* This is the Jadad scale, which rates the quality of randomized controlled trials on a scale from 0 (minimum) to 5 (maximum). The ten trials in question had a Jadad score of 1 — not good.

which sweetener participants received. The longest trial was only ten weeks long.

Think about that. This is the sum total of evidence available to us about how sweeteners impact our health. These are the trials that allow articles, books, television programs, and magazines to declare that "honey is healthy" or that "high-fructose corn syrup is harmful." Ironically, this review didn't even find the latter to be the case. The researchers found no harms from high-fructose corn syrup, and also some potential benefits from noncaloric sweeteners. That hasn't stopped many people from arguing the opposite.

Even when researchers manage to pull off higher-quality studies on dietary health, we often fall short in interpreting them. For instance, a 2015 study published in the journal *Frontiers in Nutrition* looked at eight different meta-analyses of the effect of fructose consumption on the risk of heart disease or metabolic disease (such as diabetes). It found that the average dose of fructose given to people in those trials was more than two to three times what people in the United States consume. So even if the researchers found positive results, their findings wouldn't be terribly helpful because their doses didn't represent what most people consume.

My goal is not to criticize research on sweeteners specifically. It's to highlight the sorry state of nutrition research in general. And while it's easy to point fingers at researchers and blame them for the lack of evidence about how foods affect our health, keep in mind that it's incredibly hard to do this kind of work. The reason we have to rely on small, poorly designed studies is that those are often all we have.

Study after study has shown that people, even those trying to lose weight, cannot stick to a diet for a very long period of time. These are, relatively speaking, highly motivated people who have taken it upon themselves to change what they eat. If they can't stick to a dietary regimen, how can we expect study participants who aren't as invested to follow strict instructions for months at a time?

It is very hard for researchers to find people with consistent eating habits to study. This is especially true because people often don't see immediate results from a new diet. If they think something isn't working, they're unlikely to stick with it. This has the effect of undermining research on dietary health, or at least severely limiting it. So, too, does the ready availability of all sorts of food to people participating in a study. Unlike drugs, which people can get from only a limited number of places, people can get food just about anywhere. What's more, they often don't know what's in the food they're eating. Researchers can try to get them to replace sugar packets with honey or high-fructose corn syrup, but when sweeteners are added to so many processed foods today — including pasta sauce, crackers, and soy milk — it's nearly impossible to control intake as closely as researchers need, for as long as we'd like.

Limitations like these explain why some of the most powerful studies on nutrition come from prisons or mental hospitals, where researchers can exercise more control over what people eat. But due to understandable ethical concerns about using inmates or patients as guinea pigs for experiments of any sort, these sorts of trials are rarely undertaken today.

Even if we could design better studies and get enough people to participate in them, the outcomes the general public cares about most — death and major disease — are actually pretty hard to study. To detect meaningful differences in the rates of those outcomes, researchers have to study huge numbers of people while eschewing certain groups of potential subjects, such as the elderly, altogether. (This is a choice researchers often make, because deaths from old age skew their results.) As a result, we instead focus on things we assume are linked to those bad outcomes. Many of these are process measures, such as glucose or insulin levels. They're short-term markers that we believe are related to larger, more important health outcomes, such as getting diabetes or dying. Unfortunately, changes in process measures sometimes don't translate into measurable changes in health.

Finally, as I mentioned earlier, the type of research that would allow us to make definitive connections between food and health — long-term randomized controlled trials with many participants — is extremely expensive. Most organizations that want to know more about dietary health don't have the budgets for this kind of work.

Even many food companies don't foresee a great return on investment from dietary health research. They can sell their products without "proving" that they're healthy, so why bother? (There's also a risk that the findings will be counterproductive. The study on sweeteners I discussed earlier — the one that found honey, sugar, and high-fructose corn syrup to be equally healthy — was funded by the National Honey Board, and I'm guessing that organization wasn't thrilled with the results.) What's more, even when a food industry does fund research, people tend to view the results with great skepticism, making it a losing proposition for the industry.

For all of these reasons, people who care about the health implications of their food choices have to rely on mostly small, sometimes flawed, short-term studies of nutrients and additives. The best we can do is treat the results of that research with the respect they deserve, ignoring any grandiose proclamations we might hear and examining the studies themselves whenever possible. Only in this way can we educate ourselves and those around us about what foods have been scientifically proven to have an impact on our health, and what kind of impact they can really be expected to have.

This is where *The Bad Food Bible* comes in.

HOW THIS BOOK CAN HELP

My goal in this book is to make you a more responsible consumer — both of foods and of the latest research about how foods affect your health. I also want to show you that it's okay to live a little and not be so worried about what you eat, because in many cases your fears are probably based on unfounded science. Sometimes this baseless anxiety might actually be hurting you. At the very least, it's robbing you of some potential joy.

Throughout this book, I point out when we as a society have followed the results of bad research and when we have ignored good research. As you read, try to keep a few simple ground rules in mind. Remember that human studies trump animal studies, prospective studies trump retrospective studies, and randomized controlled trials trump almost everything — except for systematic reviews and meta-analyses, which are studies of studies. (A collection of RCTs, for instance, will beat out any single RCT almost every time.)

The more you can dispense with your received wisdom about dietary health, the more you'll get out of this book. Try to carry that spirit of skepticism with you after you've finished reading it. When someone tells you to give up something you love, something that may even be healthy, try to understand where they're coming from and what arguments and evidence they're basing their claims on. If you don't understand their evidence, or if it seems suspicious, ask questions. Chances are you'll get closer to the truth than they have.

Critical thinking is an essential part of this process, because the evidence about dietary health is spotty and often contradictory, which leaves plenty of room for "creative" interpretation of the "facts." It's estimated that millions of papers get published every year. If you look hard enough, you can almost always find a study or finding to support your point of view. If you're inclined to hate meat, for instance, you can point to a study that says that for every 10% increase in your calories from animal protein, your risk of death increases 2%, while for every 3% increase in your calories from plant protein, your risk of death goes down 10%. If you're inclined to love meat, you can point to a study that says that long-term vegetarianism can lead to genetic changes that increase the risks of heart disease and cancer. In other words, you can cherry-pick. This sort of selective reasoning is how so many people get away with claiming that their beliefs about dietary health are "scientifically proven."

Nothing illustrates this better than the classic 2013 study that examined research investigating fifty common ingredients randomly selected from an ordinary cookbook. The researchers found 264 different studies that looked at forty ingredients. Their conclusion? Depending on where you look, you can find evidence that nearly everything we eat is associated with both higher *and* lower rates of cancer.

Overcoming the biases of case-control and cohort study data can be difficult. Researchers often can't get all the information they need out of a particular data set. For instance, imagine that you're studying the connection between eating meat and a particular health problem. Your data set includes only whether or not the study subjects ate meat during a certain time period and whether or not they developed that health problem. But it's possible that people who eat meat are also more likely to smoke, to be binge drinkers, to be poorer or heavier, or to come from families that have a history of heart disease or cancer. Unless all of this information about the subjects is included in the data set, you won't be able to control for it in your analysis, and you might conclude that meat is to blame for that health problem, when it's really smoking or family history.

This is a much bigger problem than most people realize. "Unhealthy" habits seem to run together. People who eat poorly are also less likely to be physically active. People who drink too much alcohol are more likely to smoke. People who abuse drugs are more likely to drink alcohol and smoke. Having money in your pocket doesn't make you healthier, but having the means to make life changes might. A simplistic study would note that richer people are healthier than poorer people, and conclude that the way to make people healthier is to buy them stocks and bonds. A better study would be able to tease out the fact that wealth is associated with health and that it allows access to certain resources that we could provide directly to people to make them healthier.

Researchers can use a variety of techniques to try to account for confounding factors, but these analytic fixes are complicated and can be problematic in themselves. That's why different meta-analyses can reach different conclusions. Unless the associations are large and unmistakable, as they are with smoking and lung cancer, it's hard to know for sure if the results you're seeing are real.

These complexities are a hallmark of health research, and you'll want to keep them in mind as you read this book. But it's also worth noting one simple fact about food: very few ingredients are categorically "bad." Food is rarely unhealthy in and of itself. More often, food becomes unhealthy when we consume too much or too little of it. The trick is to figure out how much is too much, and how little is too little.

Let me be clear: this book isn't about trying to get you to think that some foods and drinks are so good for you that you should start eating or drinking vast quantities of them. Rather, my goal is to show you that foods that have been traditionally thought of as "bad" aren't necessarily so. By marshaling all the available research about the most controversial foods, I aim to cut through the hype and the hand-wringing, and help you restore sanity to your diet.

Just as the first nutritional guidelines in the late 1800s emphasized variety and balance, this book purports to help you find equilibrium in the foods you eat. If that means abandoning the certainty that characterizes so much writing about dietary health, so be it. If it means giving you permission to indulge occasionally, so much the better.

The
BAD FOOD
BIBLE

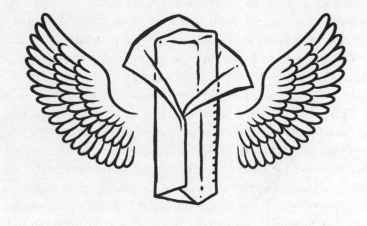

One

BUTTER

W HEN I was a kid in the 1970s, one of the biggest debates in our household had to do with what we should spread on our toast. On the one hand, butter had been a staple of the American diet for centuries, but experts recently had begun to push margarine as a healthier substitute. Butter, after all, was full of "unhealthy" saturated fat; indeed, it contained more saturated fat than just about anything else in the typical Western kitchen at the time, although cheese, cream, and other dairy products (as well as certain non-dairy animal products) came close. On the other hand, margarine was made in a lab from "healthier" vegetable fats: the unsaturated fats found in (for instance) soybean or safflower oil.

There was just one problem: at room temperature, vegetable oils are liquid. No one wants a soggy, wet piece of toast. To make margarine solid, food scientists subjected vegetable oils to a process called hydrogenation, in which hydrogen gas was mixed with the oils while exposing them to a metal catalyst and subjecting them to heat and pressure. This process created oils that were solid at room temperature and, at least at first, tested quite well in marketing research. Many people, even cardiologists, began to push margarine as a "heart healthy" substitute for butter. It became the spread of choice in the Carroll household.

Of course, today we know "hydrogenated oils" by another name: "trans fats." And now we know they're terrible for us — even worse than saturated fats. Yet the margarine-induced assault on butter continues to this day and has led people to spurn many of its saturated-fat cousins as well.

The impact of this low-fat craze on our health has been dubious, to say the least. It turns out that alternatives to saturated fats — including, but not limited to, trans fats — are not nearly as good for us as we were led to believe. And there's another wrinkle. Those saturated fats we thought were so bad for us? They actually might not be.

THE TRUTH ABOUT TRANS FATS

By the 1990s, evidence was building that trans fats carried a significant risk of coronary heart disease. Today, they've been found not only to increase levels of low-density lipoprotein (the "bad" cholesterol — more on this in chapter 3) but to also decrease levels of high-density lipoprotein (the "good" cholesterol). By both increasing LDL and decreasing HDL, trans fats have about twice the negative impact as saturated fats. And that's not all. Trans fats also increase triglycerides, fats that our body can use for energy but that are also thought to be associated with cardiovascular disease.

Unlike many other areas of nutrition science, there is some high-quality research to support the conclusion that trans fats are bad for our health. In 2006, the *New England Journal of Medicine* published a huge review article that began to sound the death knell for trans fats. The researchers conducted a meta-analysis of twelve randomized controlled trials of trans fatty acid consumption through 2005. They found that compared to eating saturated or unsaturated fats, eating trans fats significantly increased pretty much all the risk factors for coronary heart disease. Trans fats also appeared to increase the markers of inflammation in the body and decrease the effectiveness of the cells that work to keep the blood vessels clean. On a per-calorie basis, trans fats increased the risk of coronary heart disease more than any other nutrient.*

Throughout this book, I discuss how the dire warnings we hear about many ingredients seem to be overblown. I don't take that approach with trans fats, however, because the evidence against them is pretty damning.

I'm not alone in this conclusion. In recent years, artificial trans fats have been almost entirely eliminated from the American diet. Months before the study in the *New England Journal of Medicine* was published, the Food and Drug Administration ruled that companies had to start explicitly labeling how much

---

* This was true even when trans fats comprised as little as 1% to 3% of caloric intake. A 2% increase in caloric intake from trans fats was found in cohort studies to be associated with a 23% increase in the incidence of disease.

trans fats their foods contained. Fast-food retailers such as McDonald's and Burger King began eliminating artificial trans fats from their products, and the tiny amounts that remain occur naturally in meat and cheese. New York City banned them in restaurants in 2007, and the Centers for Disease Control and Prevention argued that removing trans fats from the U.S. food supply could prevent about 20,000 heart attacks a year and 7,000 deaths from cardiovascular disease. In response, the FDA issued a *Federal Register* notice announcing that the agency believes that trans fats are not "generally recognized as safe." Such a notice allows a period of time for people and businesses to comment and offer opinions and evidence as to why the determination should not result in a ban. Nothing convincing came of this, and in 2015 the FDA finalized its determination that trans fats are generally not recognized as safe.

In the butter versus margarine debate, the Carroll family should have stuck with butter. And that's not the only match in which butter appears to win out. It seems that not only are saturated fats much better for us than trans fats, but they also may not be that much worse for us than a range of other fats — including many that have been championed as "healthier" alternatives.

You read that right: butter, and the fats it contains, are not only likely to be part of a healthy diet, but they may actually be better for us than many alternatives. Frustratingly, the evidence to prove this has been out there for decades. It just hasn't been given a fair shake until very recently.

BUSTING THE "HEART HEALTHY" MYTH

In the late 1960s and early 1970s, researchers conducted what is now known as the Minnesota Coronary Experiment, a well-designed randomized controlled trial set in one nursing home and six state mental hospitals.* The study was large, involving more than 9,400 men and women between the ages of 20 and 97. At baseline — that is, before the study began — participants were getting about 18.5% of their calories from saturated fats (e.g., animal fats and butter) and about 3.8% from polyunsaturated fats. The intervention diet — the one that researchers gave to the test subjects who were not in the control group — was considered more "heart healthy" than the baseline diet because it reduced the number of calories they were consuming from saturated fats to 9.2%, and raised the amount they were getting from unsaturated fats, particularly linoleic acids (such as corn oil), to 13.2%.

The average follow-up for these participants was just under three years, meaning the modified diet had quite a long time to show its effects on the subjects' bodies.† But when researchers checked on the subjects who had been assigned the "heart healthy" diet, they found that these men and women had no decreased risk of death. If anything, mortality rates in this group seemed to have *increased,* particularly among those 65 years of age or older.

Of course, this is only one study. It involved only institutionalized patients, and only about a quarter of the participants followed the diet for more than a year. Also, the diet didn't look like what people really ate. Still, this was a large randomized controlled trial, and its results should not be marginalized or ignored.

The results of the Minnesota Coronary Experiment were not published until 2016, but in the interim more studies backed up

---

* Conducting a trial like this, in which people likely weren't given the opportunity to offer consent, is ethically questionable. I doubt that it could be done in this way today, and that's a good thing.

† This is an eternity in nutrition studies. We rarely get anything that long.

its findings that a "heart healthy" diet might actually be bad for us. For instance, an analysis of recovered data from the Sydney Diet Heart Study, a randomized controlled trial of a similar nature performed in men with a recent coronary event such as a heart attack, was published in 2013. Although the study was done from 1966 to 1973, results weren't available publicly until well into the twenty-first century. Like the Minnesota Coronary Experiment, this study found that a diet higher in unsaturated fats led to a increased rate of death from heart disease.

Looking for more clues about the connections between alternatives to saturated fats and heart disease, researchers conducted a meta-analysis of all the studies that looked at this question. Even when they amassed all the evidence, they found that more people died on linoleic acid–rich diets like the "heart healthy" one given to subjects in the Minnesota Coronary Experiment than on baseline diets that contained more saturated fats, although the results were not statistically significant.

What was significant, however, was the analysis's conclusion about the health effects of saturated fats. Even when the researchers twisted their models this way and that, and even when they included more studies of lesser quality, they couldn't find any decreased risk of dying with diets lower in saturated fats.

Other meta-analyses complicate the picture. Some support the notion that butter and other saturated fats are no better or worse for us than other kinds of fats. Others challenge it. A 2010 study, for instance, claimed to show that substituting unsaturated fats for saturated fats could reduce people's rates of coronary heart disease. So did a 2015 systematic review. By contrast, a 2014 study published in the *Annals of Internal Medicine* showed the opposite.

The dangers of saturated fats, in other words, are still up for debate — but that's not how nutrition experts have been portraying the science for decades. They've argued, loudly and stridently, that fats, especially saturated fats, are the true enemy of a healthy diet. Many of them persist in this view, despite the fact that the evidence isn't nearly as clear as their conviction might suggest.

What's going on here? Why do health experts continue to demonize saturated fats, despite a lack of data to support that conclusion? Perhaps it's for the same reason that research findings in support of saturated fats weren't available decades ago.

Remember, the results of the Minnesota Coronary Experiment weren't published until 2016, even though the data had been collected decades earlier. To be sure, it's possible that modern computer technology allowed modern-day scientists to do analyses using these data that couldn't be performed back in the 1960s and '70s, rendering publishable results that earlier would have been an unintelligible mound of facts and figures. It's also possible that researchers tried to publicize their findings at the time but were unable to get them published. And it's possible that these results were marginalized—by the scientific establishment, or even by the researchers themselves—because they didn't fit with what was considered to be the "truth" about saturated fats at the time.

The two principal investigators in the Minnesota study were Ivan Frantz and Ancel Keys,* the second of whom may be the most influential scientist ever in promoting saturated fats as the enemy of heart health. I'm not suggesting anything sinister —I'm sure that both these scientists absolutely believed that diets lower in saturated fats led to better health—but they must have been baffled that their thorough research failed to confirm their beliefs. And, like so many other researchers then and

---

* For a thorough review of the influence of Ancel Keys and his research on the history of fats in the American diet, I recommend Nina Teicholz's *The Big Fat Surprise*.

now, as they were confronting these puzzling results, they may have fallen victim to a phenomenon called *publication bias*.

Publication bias occurs when a researcher or the review board of a scientific journal decides whether to publish the results of a study based on its outcome. For instance, interesting results often get published, while uninteresting or negligible results don't; research has shown that studies with statistically significant results are more likely to be published than those without such results. Studies with a "low-priority" topic or finding—one that's less likely to make the news or change the way doctors like me practice medicine—also may be less likely to be published.

Studies that find significant associations between foods (like butter) and scary findings (like heart attacks) are more likely to be published than those that don't find such associations. Although such studies are often reported in the news media, in many cases their conclusions can't be supported by further research. When controlled trials are done to try to replicate them, researchers often find they can't. Thus, publication bias may be directly linked to the widely publicized "replication crisis" confronting modern science as a whole, and the fields of psychology and medicine in particular.

Perhaps the most common reason for publication bias is that researchers simply don't write up their work and submit it for publication. In some cases, that could be because they think it won't be accepted. But it also could be because they don't believe the results—or don't want to be associated with them. In the charged environment of nutrition research, where people's careers are built on certain hypotheses, it's harder to avoid publication bias than it is to succumb to it. There have been plenty of accusations that people who have challenged accepted nutritional beliefs have been frozen out of positions, funding, or committees.

Of course, it's not just academic reputations that are at stake; so, too, are people's lives. This is why it's important to acknowledge that the jury is still out when it comes to the health impact of saturated fats.

I know far too many people who still believe that eating fats makes you fat. This boggles the mind, given that the low-fat craze coincided so perfectly with a huge increase in overweight and obesity in the general population. What's more, many studies contradict the "fats make you fat" hypothesis. Systematic reviews of studies of all kinds of diets show that low-fat diets do not outperform other kinds of diets with respect to weight loss. A well-designed two-year study comparing a low-fat diet to a low-carb diet and the Mediterranean diet* found that while all of the diets reduced weight, the latter two outperformed the low-fat diet with respect to pounds shed.

In fact, experts now generally agree that dairy products — perhaps the most common source of saturated fats in any modern kitchen — are likely fine for you so long as you don't have too much of them. But how much dairy is too much? That depends on whom you ask.

DAIRY ISN'T THE DEVIL — BUT THAT DOESN'T MEAN YOU SHOULD OVERDO IT

If you've read my newspaper columns or watched my videos, you've likely seen me rail against the "milk-industrial complex."† I am not being hyperbolic when I call it that. Many people in the nutrition community push milk, and to a lesser

---

* The Mediterranean diet encourages eating more vegetables, olive oil (fat), nuts (fat), and protein (fish). Red wine is encouraged as well.

† I've even made reference to the "milk emperor": someday, someone is going to convince you that the milk emperor (i.e., pushers of dairy products) has no clothes.

extent dairy products in general, with an evangelism that vastly outstrips what the evidence warrants. These experts are backed up by the dairy industry, national governments, and a lot of health research to boot. But what is the basis of this mania — and how do they get away with it?

Almost no one will dispute that when a baby is born, breast milk is the best source of nutrition. All mammals nurse their young, and breast milk benefits a newborn in ways above and beyond nutrition. Breast-feeding infants until 1 to 2 years of age is optimal, according to the American Academy of Pediatrics, Institute of Medicine (now the Health and Medicine Division of the National Academies of Sciences, Engineering, and Medicine), World Health Organization, and many other renowned health groups.

Unfortunately, breast-feeding until that age is often difficult, if not impossible, for many mothers — especially those who are less well-off and have to return to work, those who go back to work by choice, and those whose children go off to preschool or day care. So we often replace human milk with the milk of cows or other animals, and we continue to consume it into adulthood. This distinguishes our species in a questionable way, if you ask me: we are the only mammals on the planet that consume milk after childhood, often in great amounts.

However, more and more evidence is surfacing that suggests milk consumption after the first few years of life has no positive effect on our health — and too much might be detrimental. This is in spite of the fact that the U.S. Department of Agriculture (USDA) recommends that adults may potentially drink 3 cups a day to meet their daily dairy requirement.

Proponents of the Paleo Diet may have a point when they argue that grown-ups don't need milk. More than 10,000 years ago, when human beings began to domesticate animals, no adults or older children consumed milk. Many people don't drink it today because they are lactose intolerant, and they do just fine without it.

According to the dairy industry, people who avoid milk are missing out on some fantastic health benefits. Milk is good for our bones, dairy producers tell us; it contains calcium and vitamin D. In the 1980s, the industry ran a popular advertising campaign using the slogan "Milk: It does a body good." But there's not much evidence for these types of claims. In fact, the research often flat out contradicts them.

One big piece of evidence in the case against milk emerged in 2011, when the *Journal of Bone and Mineral Research* published a meta-analysis examining whether milk consumption might protect against hip fractures in middle-aged and older adults. Six studies of almost 200,000 women could find no association between drinking milk and lower rates of fractures. More recent research has confirmed these findings. In a study published in 2014, researchers asked almost 100,000 men and women how much milk they had consumed as teenagers, and then followed them for more than two decades to see if milk consumption was associated with a reduced chance of hip fractures later in life. It wasn't. Another study followed more than 45,000 men and 61,000 women in Sweden age 39 or older and tracked their milk consumption as adults. These researchers found similar results, reporting that drinking milk was not associated with any protection for men, and was actually correlated with an *increased* risk of fractures in women, and an increased risk of death in both sexes. The Swedish study wasn't a randomized controlled trial, so we should not assume causality. But it's important to note that according to all these studies, drinking milk seems to have no association with benefits and may have a significant association with harm.

Even studies that have examined the specific nutrients in dairy products for possible protective effects come up short. A

2007 meta-analysis in the *American Journal of Clinical Nutrition* examined high-quality studies of how calcium intake was related to fractures. The analysis of these studies of more than 200,000 people ages 34 to 79 found no link between total calcium intake and risk of bone fractures. This meta-analysis also reviewed randomized controlled trials that examined whether calcium supplements could lower the risk of fractures. More than 6,000 middle-aged and older adults participated in these trials, in which subjects were randomly assigned to get extra calcium or a placebo. Not only did the extra calcium not reduce the rate of fractures, but the researchers were concerned that it may have *increased* the risk of hip fractures. So if your doctor (or a milk industry advertisement) is telling you to consume more dairy so as to get more calcium, you might want to ask how sure he or she is of that advice.

In the United States, dairy is often fortified with vitamin D, which many people believe has mild bone-friendly properties, as does (they think) calcium. Yet the evidence for adding vitamin D to products is sketchy. Although it is true that vitamin D is necessary for calcium absorption, and therefore for bone health, that doesn't mean most people need to consume more of it. A meta-analysis published in the *Lancet* examined the effects of vitamin D supplementation on bone mineral density in middle-aged and older adults. It found that for the most part, consuming extra vitamin D did *not* improve the bones of the spine, hip, or forearm. It did result in a statistically significant, but less clinically meaningful, increase in bone density at the top of the thighbone. As a whole, however, in the studies analyzed, vitamin D had no effect on overall body bone mineral density.

None of this should be taken to mean that people with vitamin D or calcium deficiencies shouldn't take supplements — including, perhaps, adding extra dairy to their diets. They absolutely should. But the majority of people in the United States

are not clinically deficient in these nutrients, and dairy adver-
tisements don't discriminate between people who need them
and those who don't. Nor do governments or many medical experts, for that matter.

Any recommendation to drink 3 cups of anything (besides
water) daily should raise a red flag. Milk is not a low-calorie
beverage. Even if people drink nonfat milk, 3 cups a day means
they're consuming 250 calories. Low-fat or whole milk has
even more calories. In an era when seemingly every other caloric beverage is being demonized out of concern that it's causing obesity, doesn't it seem strange that milk still gets a pass?

Politics are almost certainly at play here. The USDA's role in
promoting dairy was firmly established in the 1983 Dairy Production Stabilization Act, which made it the business of the
government to carry out a "coordinated program of promo-
tion designed to strengthen the dairy industry's position in the
marketplace and to maintain and expand domestic and foreign
markets and uses for fluid milk and dairy products." Organizations such as Dairy Management Inc., a nonprofit organization created by the U.S. government in 1995, exist to increase
dairy consumption. DMI, for instance, employed the popular
"Got Milk?" campaign to advance this agenda. Today, the vast
majority of DMI's funding for its marketing strategies comes
from dairy producers themselves. So, yes, there is a milk-industrial complex, and it doesn't seem to have your best interests at
heart.

Let me be clear: I'm not telling you never to drink milk.
Clearly, babies and toddlers are meant to drink breast milk.
They do just fine on formula and then cow's milk, too.

I'm also not telling you to believe arguments that demonize any dairy consumption at all as harmful. For instance, anyone who claims that just because our ancestors didn't drink
milk, we shouldn't either, is doing some pretty selective think-

ing. We didn't always cook our food either, but no one but a crackpot would tell you to eat all of your meat raw. Similarly, we didn't always have coffee or beer, yet there are responsible — and highly enjoyable — ways to consume both beverages. Just because we didn't eat a certain way in the past doesn't mean we can't eat that way now.

Moreover, when it comes to the overall healthiness of dairy, there's plenty of good news. Paleo Diet supporters say that dairy can cause diabetes, but a systematic review and meta-analysis of the available data showed the opposite to be true: consuming dairy seems to have a protective effect against diabetes. These supporters say that dairy can cause heart disease and death from cardiovascular events, but though the evidence is scarce, the data we do have suggest the opposite: consuming dairy seems to have a positive effect on cardiovascular health. They also say that dairy consumption can make you fat, but in truth it's not associated with significant weight gain. And they argue that eating dairy is associated with a greater risk of death from many causes, but that's not true either.

Besides, there are some pretty compelling reasons why you would want to consume milk — reasons that have more to do with pleasure than with health. What else would you put on your cereal? And cookies without milk would be unthinkable. There's nothing wrong with having an occasional glass of milk just because you like it. The same goes for the vast constellation of other dairy products. Plain yogurt is often the only thing on the breakfast buffet that isn't pretty much a dessert. Cheese, in all its forms, is delicious.

I doubt that most people fear dairy the way they do artificial sweeteners or salt or cholesterol (all subjects of later chapters in this book), but if you do, you shouldn't. The same goes for the fats these foods contain. Don't eat too much of them, and you'll be fine.

THE BOTTOM LINE

Should we be eating more polyunsaturated fats? Should we be avoiding saturated fats? It's hard to answer these questions using the available data. And knowing there's likely data out there that people haven't shared due to publication bias makes finding the truth that much more difficult.

There is one thing we *do* know about fats, however. Fat consumption does not cause weight gain. To the contrary, it might actually help us shed a few pounds.

The tide does seem to be turning in favor of saturated fats — but slowly. The halting nature of the shift is exemplified by the USDA's guidelines for nutrition, which are released every five years. These guidelines help determine how foods are labeled, set research priorities for the National Institutes of Health, and determine what foods are distributed to needy families. They are highly influential with doctors, nutritionists, policy makers, and the general public. In recent years, these guidelines have been updated to reflect some of the latest research about saturated fats. But like so much else, they get some things about saturated fats right and other things wrong.

Before the USDA issues its five-year nutritional report, its Dietary Guidelines Advisory Committee reviews the relevant — and hopefully new — research and recommends changes from the previous report. In 2015, the committee took several strong positions on saturated fats, some good and some debatable. For instance, they concluded that replacing saturated fats with polyunsaturated fats seems to reduce the risk of cardiovascular events and mortality. Based on the evidence I've reviewed, I'm not nearly as sure about this as they are. They also acknowledged that replacing fats with carbohydrates, which many people did after fats in general were discouraged in previous reports, does not lower health risks. On that, we agree. (As I discuss in chapter 9, there's no reason for most people to be increasing their carbohydrate consumption.) The committee concluded that saturated fats should be limited to 10% of a person's total caloric intake; all other fats should be polyunsaturated, such as those from non-hydrogenated vegetable oils (olive oil, corn oil, or sunflower oil).

Besides the warning against replacing dietary fats with carbs, there is one other area on which the committee and I (and many other health experts) agree: there aren't any good reasons to restrict unsaturated fats — the kind you get from eating nuts, seeds, or olives. In fact, there's rapidly growing evidence that you should be *seeking out* these fats. They're key components of the Mediterranean diet, which has been vindicated time and again for preventing a host of health problems, mostly cardiovascular ones.

It's hard to overemphasize what a dramatic shift in thinking this is. Twenty years ago, many people were dismissive of low-carb diets. Instead, people were flocking to low-fat foods. When Gary Taubes published his groundbreaking *New York Times Magazine* article "What If Fat Doesn't Make You Fat?" in 2002, many experts disagreed with him quite vociferously. Twelve years later, when Nina Teicholz published *The Big Fat Surprise,* she took to task many of those people and organizations that had led the way in demonizing fats. For this, and for other pieces she's written, many in the nutrition community pilloried her.

I've written, sometimes a bit critically, about both Taubes and Teicholz. But I think we agree on much more than we disagree on. The evidence against fats is fading fast, and the data supporting the reasonable consumption of them seem to be on the rise. It's likely that both Taubes and Teicholz will be owed many apologies in the future.

Bottom line? The evidence in favor of a low-fat diet is very thin, whereas the evidence for the benefits of certain fats is mounting. To be sure, trans fats appear to be terrible for you, but thankfully they've been largely removed from our diets already, thanks to government regulations and self-regulation by food companies. Saturated fats may be bad for you in large amounts, but that issue is far from settled. Unsaturated fats seem to have few negative health consequences, and trying to limit them — especially if you're replacing those calories with carbohydrates — is a bad idea.

So take heart: a bit of butter — or cream, or animal fat — won't hurt you, especially if you're using it to season vegetables, fish, or other components of a healthy diet.

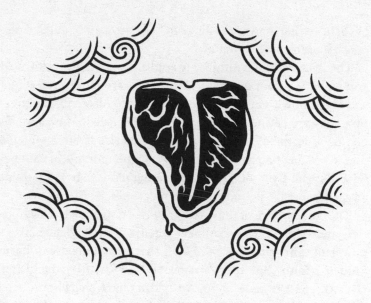

Two

MEAT

I T'S possible that no food has been attacked as widely or as loudly in the past few decades as meat. Advocates of meatless diets push them for lots of different reasons, perhaps the biggest being the claim that they can reduce the risk of cancer. One of the leading voices in this school of thought was the Japanese scholar Michio Kushi, who promoted his macrobiotic (and meatless) way of life in books such as *The Cancer Prevention Diet,* first published in 1983. But he's not alone. Many people believe that a meatless diet can help stave off a range of diseases, thereby prolonging life.

There's something intuitively appealing about the anti-meat argument. Without question, Westerners are more overweight and obese now than they were in the past.* Also without question, they are eating more meat than they have in recent memory. Back in the 1950s, for instance, Americans ate about 138 pounds of meat a year on average, with 107 pounds of that being red meat. By 2000, they were eating more than 195 pounds a year, almost 114 pounds of it red meat.

The coincidence of these two trends — rising meat consumption and expanding waistlines — seems at first glance like a powerful affirmation of the claim that eating meat can harm human health. But there's a problem with this conclusion. Over the past decade or so, Americans have sharply reduced their meat consumption. In 2012, they were down to about 132 pounds a year — 6 pounds below the average in the 1950s. More dramatically, red meat consumption had dropped to 71 pounds, 36 pounds below the 1950s level, as Americans switched to more "white meat" such as chicken.

If meat, especially red meat, is all that bad for you, the United States should be seeing massive declines in obesity rates or deaths from cardiovascular disease. But Americans are not getting any less fat, nor does their decline in meat consumption seem to be lowering their likelihood of dying from heart disease, at least not when you look carefully at the research. It shows that even purported links aren't as strong as they might appear at first glance. Rates of deaths from heart disease have been down over the past few decades, but that is likely due to lower smoking rates, better emergency response systems, ad-

---

* In general, overweight is defined as having a body mass index (BMI) between 25 and 30, and obese is having a BMI of 30 or higher.

vances in medications and procedures, and increased public health measures to create healthier environments and encourage more physical activity.

When it comes to obesity and heart disease, lowering the amount of meat in one's diet does not seem to be a silver bullet. Yet calls for reducing meat consumption are just as loud today as they were back in the early 1980s, when Michio Kushi published his book. Meat's opponents often back up their claims with scientific studies that appear to show a causal link between meat consumption and health problems, and blame meat's saturated fat and high protein content for these effects. But, as with so many other warnings about "bad" foods, condemnations of meat are likely more definitive than they should be. In fact, if certain people follow this advice, it may actually harm them.

WHO SAYS MEAT WILL KILL YOU?

You have to bend the truth — or at least do some pretty selective reasoning — to make a scientific case that meat is bad for you.

For instance: In 2015, the physician and diet guru Dean Ornish wrote an editorial in the *New York Times* titled "The Myth of High-Protein Diets." In it, he argued that plant-based diets are healthier than those containing meat. "An optimal diet for preventing disease is a whole-foods, plant-based diet that is naturally low in animal protein, harmful fats and refined carbohydrates," he wrote. "What that means in practice is little or no red meat."

Ornish is a major proponent of a low-fat diet, so the fact that he was urging readers to reduce or eliminate their meat consumption wasn't surprising in and of itself. But his use of the data was.

In his op-ed, Ornish cited research that he claimed showed that eating meat was more likely to make you die at a younger age. He mentioned one particular study, published in 2014, that followed thousands of people over time to determine whether what they ate might be linked to the chances of their getting a disease or dying. As Ornish described it, this research found that increased protein intake was associated with large increases in mortality rates from all diseases, with high increases in the chances of death from cancer or diabetes.

The thing is, that's not exactly what the study showed. Overall, the researchers found no association between protein consumption and death from all causes, or from cardiovascular disease or cancer individually, when everyone over age 50 was considered.* In other words, the study suggested that when all adults are considered together, eating meat isn't bad for them.

So how do people like Ornish get away with saying the research says otherwise? The "scary" finding they like to cite was found only among people ages 50 to 65. In that group, eating more protein was associated with an increased risk of death, especially from cancer or diabetes. But in people age 65 or older, the opposite was true: eating more protein was associated with lower levels of all-cause and cancer-specific mortality. As the researchers themselves put it when summing up their findings, "These results suggest that low protein intake during middle age followed by moderate to high protein consumption in old adults may optimize healthspan and longevity."

In this instance, both Ornish and the researchers whose work he was citing probably overstated the findings of this study. If you truly believe that it proves what meat detractors say, that

---

* The researchers did find a statistically significant association between the consumption of protein and death from diabetes, but they warned that the number of people in the analysis was so small that any results should be viewed with caution.

meat may kill people under the age of 65, then you must also think that meat may save people age 65 or older. Not many diet experts would tell you that's the case, let alone recommend that you reshape your diet because of it. Furthermore, this study put anyone who got 20% or more of their calories from protein in the "high protein" group. Almost all of the guidelines and recommendations I can find do not consider that amount of protein "high." In fact, according to USDA guidelines — which do not constitute a high-protein diet — Americans should get 10% to 35% of their calories from protein.

This is a great example of how research can get twisted. Does this study show that eating more meat is more likely to make you die? Only if you agree with the researchers' definition of "high protein" and restrict the analysis to a certain artificially divided population — this is, if you make your case by selectively picking certain factors.*

Sadly, this is only one example of this phenomenon. Over and over again, researchers and health experts cherry-pick evidence to back up their belief that people should eat less meat. Their intentions may be good. As Ornish himself points out in the conclusion of his *New York Times* essay, eating less meat can lessen the impact of animal farming on the environment and free up more grain for hungry people. But that doesn't change the fact that from a health standpoint, the case against meat isn't nearly as clear-cut as he and other anti-meaters claim.

There's another problem with this anti-meat logic. "Meat" is a very broad category. A pork chop, a hamburger, and a piece of scrod all qualify as meat. But the nutritional content of meat varies wildly based on the cut, the animal it comes from, and

---

* If I wanted to cherry-pick myself, I might point you to a 2013 study that used the same National Health and Nutrition Examination Survey data to conclude that meat consumption is *not* associated with mortality at all. But let's avoid cherry-picking.

many other factors. Are these different kinds of meat good for you or bad for you? It depends on whom you ask—and where you look.

FISH IS GOOD FOR YOU—NO BONES ABOUT IT

All meat isn't created equal. Even people who argue that meat isn't good for you usually aren't thinking of fish or seafood. Those types of "meat" aren't high in saturated fats and aren't typically the focus of warnings about animal consumption, unless those warnings are coming from macrobiotic proponents like Michio Kushi. In fact, as we saw in the previous chapter, many evidence-based diets, such as the Mediterranean diet, advocate for fish consumption in addition to fruits, vegetables, and oils high in unsaturated fats, such as olive oil.

Even so, in recent years fish has been added to the list of panic-inducing foods alongside other kinds of meat. Tuna, for example, has become a concern for many health-conscious individuals. In this case, however, they aren't worried about something intrinsic to the nutritional content of fish. Rather, they're fretting about mercury.

Mercury is a metal that exists in a liquid state at room temperature. It used to be the silver stuff you'd see in thermometers, but it's not commonly used for that purpose anymore because it's poisonous. In high enough doses, it can cause brain damage in kids and even adults.

Mercury is found in small but rising amounts in seawater. Of course, humans normally don't drink seawater, but fish do, and over time they absorb mercury from it. Once it's in their bodies, it's very hard to get rid of, and as fish grow, so do their levels of mercury.

Fish that live longer have higher levels of mercury, and the bigger the fish, the bigger the problem. When big fish eat little fish, they also eat the mercury in their bodies. Large, long-lived fish such as sharks and swordfish have the highest levels of mercury.

Let me be clear: mercury is bad for people, and especially for pregnant women. But that does not mean that people in general, and pregnant women in particular, should avoid fish entirely, as some experts argue. In regard to pregnant women, the only way you can justify that conclusion is if you misinterpret the available research on the effects of mercury on pregnant women and their children. One way to measure mercury levels in people is to check how much there is in their hair. A study published in the *American Journal of Preventive Medicine* in 2005 claimed that for every 1 microgram of mercury per gram detectable in a pregnant woman's hair, an infant might see a decrease of 0.7 point in his or her IQ. But what are the practical implications of such a decrease, and how much fish would a woman have to consume to see this effect?

Upon closer inspection, these findings are much less dramatic than they appear at first glance. For one thing, this decrease in IQ would be pretty much negligible in everyday life. Given that 90 percent of pregnant women in the United States have no more than 1.4 micrograms of mercury per gram of their hair, it's hard to imagine that anyone would experience more than a point or two difference in IQ at most from this source. Note that the median value of the mercury levels in women was 0.2 microgram per gram of hair, which is barely noticeable.

In addition, many other studies suggest mothers who eat more fish during pregnancy tend to have *more intelligent* babies. Researchers who looked at overall fish consumption found that higher maternal fish intake was associated with smarter kids. They found that women who had lower mercury levels but ate fish two or more times a week had infants with the highest cognitive scores. Some scientists attribute this to the omega-3 fatty acids in fish. But here's the problem: fish that have high levels of these wonderful fatty acids — tuna, for instance — also tend to have high levels of mercury, simply because they live longer and grow bigger.

These were all observational studies, so the findings aren't nearly as reliable as they would be if they were from experimental studies. But that's all we have to go on.*

Taken together, these studies suggest that pregnant women should stick to fish that are high in omega-3 fatty acids and low in mercury (think salmon, herring, sardines) and avoid fish that are low in omega-3 fatty acids and high in mercury (think grouper, orange roughy, canned tuna). Really, the same general guidelines apply to women who aren't pregnant, men, and children. Maximizing omega-3 fatty acids while minimizing mercury is never a bad idea.

Unfortunately, the panic over mercury has led some people to avoid fish entirely. That's almost always a bad idea.

The best evidence we have indicates that fish is good for us on the whole, regardless of its mercury content. In 2006, two researchers published the results of a study in which they reviewed all the available evidence about eating fish but focused on four main questions: (1) how much consuming fish or fish oil influences the risk of heart disease; (2) how much consuming mercury in fish and fish oil influences early neurodevelopment; (3) how much consuming mercury in fish influences heart disease and neurologic outcomes in adults; and (4) how much consuming dioxins and polychlorinated biphenyls in fish influences other health effects. They found that for most

---

* No one is going to conduct a randomized controlled trial of fish with different levels of mercury and omega-3 fatty acids to see whether eating them makes babies subsequently smarter or not. That would be unethical, not to mention terribly impractical. So this may be the best type of evidence we're going to get.

healthy adults, the benefits of eating fish outweighed the risks. For pregnant women, too, the benefits of *modest* fish intake (with the exception of a few species, as previously noted) outweighed the risks.

Most other studies of fish consumption and human health support these conclusions. In a number of studies, fish consumption has been associated with a reduced risk of esophageal cancer and ovarian cancer. It has not been associated with an increased risk of colon cancer. It has been found to be linked to a lower risk of developing diabetes. The Mediterranean diet, which recommends eating lots of fish, has been shown to prevent many undesirable cardiovascular outcomes, including heart attacks and death. Also to its credit, the Mediterranean diet is supported by randomized controlled trials, the strongest type of research to prove causation.

Anyone who says that fish is bad for you is either unfamiliar with the evidence or is using it selectively. As with other foods, you should think for yourself and eat accordingly.

"WHITE MEAT" IS MOSTLY FINE, TOO

Most research indicates that chicken and other poultry are healthy. There doesn't seem to be nearly as much research on poultry as there is on other types of meat, but if you dig deep, you can find some.

For starters, the nutritional components of poultry are favorable. Its protein is easily digested and not high in calories. Its fat is mostly unsaturated (about two-thirds) and is located mainly in the skin, which can easily be removed.

Eating poultry has *not* been associated with cancer, and, like fish, it has been associated with a decreased risk of developing diabetes. Studies of mortality from cardiovascular disease, cancer, or even all causes lumped together have detected no harmful effects of eating poultry. Even breast cancer, a commonly cited concern regarding so many foods, doesn't appear to be associated with poultry, according to a meta-analysis of prospective (higher-quality) studies. If prostate cancer is your concern, there is some evidence showing that eating more poultry is associated with lower rates of the progression of the disease and of its recurrence.

In 2009, researchers from the National Cancer Institute published results from the National Institutes of Health–AARP Diet and Health Study, a cohort study of more than half a million people ages 50 to 71. They collected a ton of data about the people themselves, how much and what they ate, and whether they exercised, smoked, or drank. The researchers then used these data to try to quantify whether meat intake was related to mortality. They found that those who consumed the most white meat had lower rates of death overall and specifically from cancer compared with those who consumed the least.

The pork industry would like us to believe that meat from pigs is in the same camp as poultry. In fact, its entire "The Other White Meat" campaign was an argument that pork is more like chicken than steak. With respect to color, that is sometimes the case. But health experts mostly care about the saturated fat content, and by that metric, pork isn't *quite* as healthy as the industry would have you believe.

Generally speaking, pork's saturated fat content is somewhere between that of poultry and red meat. But that's not a hard-and-fast rule. A lean piece of pork might have less saturated fat than a chicken leg with the skin on, even though chicken contains more unsaturated fat than saturated fat. Another cut of pork might have more saturated fat than a piece of lean red meat. As I explained in chapter 1, the jury is still out on how saturated fats affect our health. Most of the evidence seems to indicate that large quantities of saturated fats are bad for us but that moderate amounts are fine. Basically, this means that we can have as much lean meat as we want, but we should save meat with a lot of fat for a special occasion.

A study published in 2012 looked at 164 overweight but otherwise healthy adults who claimed to eat "low" amounts of pork. Half of them were randomized to substitute about 1 kilogram of lean pork a week into their diets in place of mainly chicken or beef. The researchers then followed both groups for six months. They found that compared with the control group, those in the pork-fed group lost more weight and fat. Given that this study was funded by Australian Pork Limited and the Pork Cooperative Research Centre, these results should be taken with a hefty grain of salt.

Another randomized controlled trial, funded by one of these groups and performed by many of the same scientists, randomized overweight men and women to consume 1 kilogram per week of lean pork, chicken, or beef for three months each (in addition to an otherwise unrestricted diet) to see how their weight and fat levels changed. The researchers did not observe any significant differences between the control and study groups on either metric.

A third randomized controlled trial (also funded by Australian Pork Limited) randomized young women to one of three groups: extra pork, extra iron, or a control diet. They found that the young women in the pork group ate less energy-dense, nutrient-poor foods (i.e., "bad" foods) and more fruit.

I cite these studies not because I feel they are definitive — they're almost certainly not — but rather because they are randomized controlled trials, albeit ones that were conducted for only short periods of time and that are clearly fraught with some serious conflicts of interest. Unfortunately, as I noted in the introduction, when it comes to food, sometimes companies are the only organizations that seem willing to fund interventional studies.

A systematic review published in 2013 found that people's glucose and insulin responses after a pork meal were no different than after a meal consisting of beef, shrimp, or mixed sources of protein. However, processed pork meats, such as ham, were more concerning in a limited number of the studies reviewed.

A fourteen-year cohort study in the Netherlands found that older women who consumed more pork (or chicken!) seemed to have slightly higher body mass indexes at the end of the study, but the results weren't that striking and weren't seen in men.

Overall, my review of the literature found that for the most part, studies have failed to show an association between eating lean pork products and bad outcomes with regard to cancer and heart disease. This ignores the fact that many pork products are processed or fatty (think sausage, bacon, pork belly, ham). More on those later in this chapter.

THE MEAT YOU'VE BEEN WAITING FOR: RED MEAT

Fish, poultry, and pork all come in for their share of criticism, but the real bad guy in the meat wars is red meat. Many people believe that eating red meat can kill you, and they may even be able to cite research to back up their beliefs. For instance, they may cite a 2014 meta-analysis that examined all the prospective trials that existed and found that people in the highest consumption group of all red meat had a 29% relative increase in all-cause mortality compared with those in the lowest consumption group. But even this rigorous study (remember, meta-analysis is one of the most reliable ways researchers have to process data) has a lot of gray areas, and it's usually such weak spots that anti-meaters exploit to make their point.

It's important to keep in mind, however, that most scientific studies don't come out and say "Meat will kill you." They contain statistics, definitions, qualifications, and lots of data. In many of the studies examined in this meta-analysis, for instance, people in the highest consumption group were defined as eating one to two servings of red meat a day. The people in the lowest group ate about two servings a week. If you're eating multiple servings of red meat *a day,* then, yes, you might want to cut back. But if you're eating only a couple of servings a week, you're probably doing great.

Of course, not all red meat is created equal. Meat is graded by the USDA on its nutritional content. Lean cuts of beef are those that contain less than 10 grams of fat, 4.5 grams of saturated fat, and 95 mg of cholesterol per 3.5-ounce serving. Extra-lean cuts have less than 5 grams of fat, 2 grams of saturated fat, and 95 mg of cholesterol per serving. Cuts such as eye of the round, sirloin, and top and bottom rounds tend to be leaner than others. Ground beef is defined similarly based on the cuts from which it is made.

Meat is also graded on its marbling, or how much fat is integrated in the muscle. Marbled fat is nearly impossible to trim, so if you're going for fat content, you'll want to pick "choice" or "select" cuts rather than "prime." If, however, you're going for flavor, you'll want to choose a fattier cut, such as a porterhouse, T-bone, or rib-eye steak. Even a well-marbled filet will have too much fat to be labeled "lean." Sadly, the better cuts have the most fat.

I don't eat that much steak — at most, maybe once every other week. Because of that, when I do eat it, I splurge. My wife, Aimee, has mastered pan-searing a perfect medium-rare filet, and everyone in my house loves it. Maybe once a week, I enjoy a perfect cheeseburger. I never worry about the fat content, because this level of consumption places me at the low end in most studies.

The constant drumbeat of warnings about red meat appears to have reshaped our eating habits. Americans, on average, eat less red meat today than at any time since the 1970s. We're doing a bit better in our consumption of vegetables, too. Unfortunately, those changes don't seem to have improved our health. It turns out that we're also eating more carbohydrates — and that could be, in part, due to our obsession with avoiding red meat. (See chapter 9 for a full discussion of carbs — and of how harmful it can be to consume too many of them.)

THE CANCER MYTH

Rather than renouncing their overblown anti-meat rhetoric, some health experts are doubling down on their scare tactics. Consider the World Health Organization's 2015 Q&A about processed meat and red meat. Based on epidemiologic data, as well as four hundred studies on processed meat and cancer and seven hundred on red meat, the WHO's International Agency for Research on Cancer declared that processed meat "causes cancer" and that red meat is "probably carcinogenic." Relying on a meta-analysis of cohort studies published in *PLOS ONE* in 2011, the WHO concluded that consuming an extra serving of processed meat each day would increase your risk of colon cancer by 18%.

Words like "causes" and "probably causes" are some of the strongest in health researchers' vocabularies. In this case, the language is likely too strong. It turns out that in compiling their report, the good folks at the WHO fell prey to a common prob-

lem in statistical research: confusing association with causation. They saw a relative increase of a health risk in some studies and interpreted that as evidence that the factor they were
interested in — processed or red meat consumption — was responsible for that increase, without any evidence proving a
causal link.

If you want to prove causality, the best type of study is a randomized controlled trial. Although these trials are all too rare
when it comes to nutrition research, they do exist for red meat
consumption, including some trials that have examined its potential links to cancer. The Polyp Prevention Trial, for example,
randomly assigned some of its 2,000 participants who were at
high risk for cancer to a diet high in fiber, fruits, and vegetables
and low in fats and meat. After four years of following this diet,
cancer rates were unchanged. The Women's Health Initiative,
which involved almost 50,000 women, also randomized some
of the participants to a "healthier" diet of increased fruits, vegetables, and grains and decreased fats and meat. After following these women for eight years, researchers still couldn't show
that eating less meat reduced the risk of colorectal cancer.

You can argue that these studies are insufficient — that we
need to watch trial participants for longer periods of time or
study more people. But if researchers can't find a difference in
tens of thousands of people over eight years, it may be time to
admit that even if there is a relationship between processed or
red meat consumption and cancer, it must be pretty small.

Ironically, even though solid experimental research has not
shown processed or red meat to be harmful so far, the WHO's
2015 warning makes bigger and better trials less likely to occur
in the future. After all, if the WHO has declared that processed
meat causes cancer, how can we ethically randomize people to
eat it?

It's worth keeping in mind that even big international organizations like the WHO are just as prone to confirmation bias as individual experts. For example, twenty-five years ago the WHO ruled that coffee was "possibly carcinogenic," and despite the huge amount of evidence to the contrary that was published over the years, the agency didn't change its ruling until 2016. (See chapter 8 for more on this.) It's also worth looking at the organization's warnings about processed and red meat in the context of other, similar proclamations it's made over the years. Of the 1,001 substances the WHO had evaluated as of April 2017, only *one* was labeled "probably not carcinogenic to humans."*

For the sake of argument, though, let's take the WHO at its word that an actual link exists between processed meat consumption and cancer. What's missing from its discussion is any talk about the magnitude of the risk. The WHO warning only delivered an opinion on *whether* a link exists, not *how strong* it is. Again, this is in keeping with other WHO cancer assessments. For instance, the organization has effectively lumped together in the same category ("carcinogenic to humans") tobacco smoke, which has an unequivocal and large risk, and alcohol, which likely has some benefits and a rather small risk of cancer when not abused. The same goes for the sun, which surely can cause skin cancer, but which isn't something anyone would tell you to avoid altogether.

Based on the *PLOS ONE* meta-analysis, the WHO reported that for each 50 grams of processed meat eaten daily, the risk of colon cancer goes up by 18%. That sounds scary, but that's a relative risk increase, not an absolute risk increase.

The distinction between relative risk and absolute risk is hugely important when it comes to gauging health research. To see why, consider the following scenario: Say I am trying to

---

* If you're curious, it's caprolactam, and it's a component of nylon fibers.

compare the effectiveness of two cancer drugs. One has been shown to decrease patients' risk of dying from 12% to 6%. The relative risk reduction of taking this drug would be 50% (6% being half of 12%), while the absolute risk reduction would be 6% (the number of percentage points the patients' risk has decreased). The other drug might offer the same relative risk reduction of 50%, from 0.7% to 0.35%, but a much smaller absolute risk reduction, only 0.35%. Although these two drugs have the same relative risk reduction, the first drug is much more powerful than the second.

The media likes to focus on relative risk increases. That's because they are always bigger and scarier than absolute risk increases. Bigger and scarier makes for better news stories, but not better or more informed health decisions. For those, absolute risk matters much more.

Because relative risk is such a slippery metric, I decided to see what the WHO warning about processed meat would mean for me in practical terms. First, I figured out my background risk of colon cancer by going to the National Cancer Institute's colorectal cancer risk assessment calculator and plugging in all my information. Although I'm not yet 50, I had to give that as my age because the calculator doesn't work for people younger than that. I found that the average lifetime risk of a 50-year-old for developing colorectal cancer is 6%, but my odds are better than that because I'm not obese, I eat plenty of vegetables, I exercise regularly, and I don't have a family history of colon cancer. Based on those factors, 50-year-old me has a 2.4% lifetime risk of getting colon cancer.

Now, recall that the WHO warning says that for every 50 grams of processed meat I eat daily, my relative risk of colon cancer goes up by 18%. This means that if I decided today to start eating an extra three pieces of bacon *every day for the next thirty years,* my lifetime risk of getting colon cancer might go from 2.4% to 2.8%. In terms of absolute risk, that's an increase of less than 0.5%. Put another way, if 250 people like me made the decision to start eating that much more bacon, one of them *might* get cancer, and the other 249 would be unaffected.

That's not nearly as scary as the WHO would have you believe. Even with all that processed meat (and I can't see adding an additional three pieces of bacon to my diet every day for the rest of my life), a lifetime risk of less than 3% is still pretty small. Eating bacon occasionally, which is more likely, is not going to measurably affect my lifetime risk.

THE BOTTOM LINE

With meat as with everything else, moderation is key. If you're eating multiple portions of processed meat a day, you may see some small decrease in your lifetime risk of getting cancer by cutting back on it. Maybe. But if you're like most people I know, enjoying bacon or prosciutto or some other processed meat a couple of times a week, the WHO's concerns shouldn't cause a change in your eating habits. Nor should any other media reports equating meat consumption with a higher risk of death.

What's more, if you're eating unprocessed fish, chicken, or pork, and not existing on it as your sole means of sustenance, you likely have little to worry about. Even if you're eating unprocessed red meat a couple of times a week, it's hard to find good evidence that you should change your ways.

Meat, eaten in moderation and in a thoughtful way, isn't going to kill you. Nor is avoiding it completely going to save you. Michio Kushi promoted the macrobiotic diet for his entire life. He got colon cancer at age 81 and died from pancreatic cancer seven years later.

Since I did the research for this chapter, I've stopped wor-

rying about ordering a nice, big steak once in a while in a restaurant. I eat fish all the time. I've gone back to eating buffalo
wings without guilt. And when anyone I know travels to Philadelphia, my wife and I give them a cooler to bring back frozen cheesesteaks prepared by our favorite restaurant there. We
serve them to our friends — even those who normally eschew
meat — and they all eat them. No one can pass up a Mama's
Cheesesteak.*

---

* I was born and raised in Philadelphia. We take our cheesesteaks seriously. If you're in Philadelphia, go to Mama's Pizzeria. Tell them I sent you. You won't be disappointed.

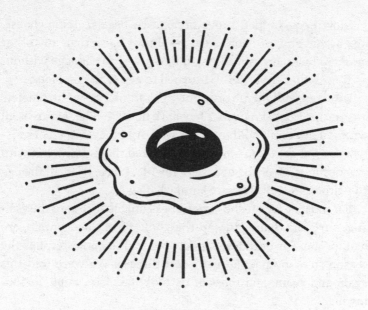

Three

EGGS

W HEN I was growing up, my family generally didn't qualify as "healthy eaters." We didn't just indulge in most of the foods covered in this book; we *over-indulged.*

But not when it came to cholesterol. My parents were rabidly anti-egg. They were anti-shrimp. They were anti-butter. Anything they thought might lead to increased cholesterol was verboten.

I love eggs. In fact, I love breakfast—bagels, cream cheese, lox, bacon, and, of course, eggs—almost more than any other meal. So in an attempt to try to find a way to eat eggs without getting all that cholesterol, I turned to egg-white omelets.

Disagree with me if you want, but I think egg-white omelets are a crime against nature. They have no taste. The texture is all wrong. They don't hold together well. And they don't feel satisfying as you eat them—or after. I choked them down, but with great protest. Over the course of my life, I have tried all the egg substitutes as well. They're similarly flawed.

For most of my life, however, I was unable to ignore the "science" arguing that eggs, and the cholesterol they contain, are bad for me. For decades, experts pointed to cholesterol as the reason so many people had heart disease. We were told this again and again, and most of us took it at face value, including me.

Finally, though, those egg-white omelets got the better of me. I began to dig deeper into the scientific literature on cholesterol. And what I found complicates the dire picture the medical establishment painted for us. To be sure, certain kinds of cholesterol really are bad for us. But not all. Some, we actually need. But which is which?

GOOD CHOLESTEROL VERSUS BAD CHOLESTEROL

Cholesterol is a fat-like substance that occurs naturally in animal tissue. Like fats, it's a type of waxy, water-repellent compound called a lipid, and many foods that are high in saturated fats—dairy products, for instance—are also high in cholesterol.

Cholesterol hurts us by getting into our blood, where it causes heart disease—still the biggest killer in the industrial world. When you have too much cholesterol in your blood, it can stick to the walls of your arteries. These are the vessels that carry blood away from your heart and to the rest of your body, and you want them to be nice and smooth so that the oxygen, nutrients, and other vital resources transported by your blood can reach the rest of your body without difficulty. Your arteries contain a thin layer of cells known as the endothelium, which helps to maintain the smoothness of the vessels.

High levels of cholesterol, as well as other factors, can lead to damage of the endothelium. That allows cholesterol to bind to, and even start to enter, the walls of your blood vessels. Your body responds by sending in other cells to try to fix the problem, but that can lead to more problems. Over time, this whole mess solidifies and becomes plaque; your soft arteries start to become hard and stiff, and they can even become blocked. When your arteries become so blocked that you can't get blood to where it needs to go, that part of your body can develop ischemia, a fancy word for "suffocation." When the blockage prevents enough blood and oxygen from getting to your heart, you have a heart attack. When it prevents blood and oxygen from getting to your brain, you have a stroke. None of these things are good, to say the least.

My father, now retired, was a general and thoracic surgeon. Growing up, I got to hear about cardiovascular disease all the time. When I was in fourth grade, I did a presentation on atherosclerosis — the medical term for plaque buildup on artery walls — complete with real X-rays that I brought to class as visual aids. Yes, I was a bit of a nerd.

For someone raised to care about heart health, as I was, the argument against cholesterol made sense. Heart disease is prevalent, and it's horrible. Atherosclerosis is a major part of it, and cholesterol in your blood is a major part of that. Eating cholesterol must contribute to the problem, right? It has to lead to more cholesterol in your blood. That's what the experts told us, and it took very little effort for them to convince us that we should avoid cholesterol at any cost.

But here's the thing: many factors have been linked to heart disease, and cholesterol is just one of them. In fact, we *need* cholesterol. It's not poison. The liver makes about 1,000 mg of it a day, because it's absolutely necessary to create certain vitamins and hormones, build parts of your cells, and help digest and move fat around your body. All told, our bodies synthesize three to four times more cholesterol than most people eat in a day. Clearly, it's important.

There are actually two kinds of cholesterol in your body. Low-density lipoprotein (LDL) is the kind that's been implicated in causing atherosclerosis; we think of this as the "bad" cholesterol. High-density lipoprotein (HDL) is the "good" cholesterol; the more of it you have, the better you do.

When you get your blood tested for cholesterol levels, the laboratory calculates a number of things. The first is likely your total cholesterol. This is the amount of LDL and HDL combined in your blood. It's also the number that most people quote and remember when they're talking about whether their cholesterol is "high." But the lab also measures the individual types, LDL and HDL, as well as triglycerides. Triglycerides are fats that circulate in your bloodstream and that your body can use for energy. High triglyceride levels also are linked to heart disease.

All of these are important, but the exact goals — specifically, the right amount of cholesterol you need — are debatable. For instance, my total cholesterol is borderline high. But my HDL levels are also high, so I don't think my "high cholesterol" is necessarily a bad thing. Because I have more good cholesterol and less bad cholesterol, the total cholesterol doesn't matter that much. But this view is somewhat controversial. Some people rely on the ratio between LDL and HDL when determining their overall health. Others focus on total cholesterol. Still others look at some combination of total cholesterol, HDL, and LDL. No one knows exactly which we should choose.

Further, it's still unclear as to whose cholesterol levels should be monitored: everyone's or only those of people in specific groups. For a long time, we tested just adults at high risk. Then we started screening pretty much all adults. In recent years, there have been calls to begin screening children as well, although there is a lot of opposition to that idea. We don't necessarily know what to do with kids once we test them. For instance, we don't know whether kids with high cholesterol will become adults at high risk. We don't know whether intervening with them will make a difference when they are adults. We also don't know whether there are long-term implications of putting kids on cholesterol-lowering drugs, potentially for decades.

In short, when it comes to cholesterol, there are many open questions. But what generally hasn't been contested, at least not publicly, is the idea that we should avoid cholesterol in our food. Which is a pity, because the cholesterol you eat has less to do with your cholesterol levels than you might think.

DIETARY CHOLESTEROL IS NOT THE PROBLEM

For a long time, guidelines like those from the USDA told us that we should limit our intake of cholesterol to no more than 300 mg a day. That's not a lot. Just one egg has about 220 mg of cholesterol. A two-egg omelet would, therefore, be a bad idea. Forget a three-egg omelet. One egg might be okay so long as we really tried to limit our cholesterol intake for the rest of the day.

Cholesterol warnings have been in effect since the 1960s. Since 1994, the U.S. government has required food companies to report cholesterol values on nutrition labels so that we can make more informed choices.

We listened to the warnings. We cut out eggs. We cut out meat. We cut out shrimp. Today, the average adult male in the United States consumes only about 340 mg of cholesterol a day, and many experts complain that's still too much.

All of these guidelines and recommendations are based on the assumption — a big one — that eating cholesterol raises blood cholesterol levels. And because it seems pretty clear that high levels of LDL cholesterol in the blood are related to the development of atherosclerosis, and that atherosclerosis is related to the risk of health problems such as heart attack and stroke, people who study this sort of thing have told us to minimize the amount of cholesterol we consume as much as possible. But the fact remains that this advice is based on an assumption.

We could, of course, design studies to test the hypothesis that dietary cholesterol affects blood cholesterol levels, and indeed researchers have done this. For instance, a 2004 study randomized participants into two groups. One group was given the equivalent of more than three eggs a day for thirty days, and the other received a placebo. Then they switched the groups, so that those who had been consuming the eggs started to get the placebo, and those who had been receiving the placebo started to eat the eggs. To see how egg consumption affected their blood, the researchers measured the participants' cholesterol after the first thirty days and then after the second thirty days. What they found is that about 70% of people are what we call "hyporesponders" to dietary cholesterol. This means that their blood cholesterol levels have almost no relationship to how much cholesterol they eat.

The results of just this one study might not move you, but there have been many others like it. In 2013, researchers published a systematic review of studies over the previous decade that examined the link between cholesterol consumed and cholesterol levels. Twelve met the review study's criteria, and seven of the twelve controlled for background diet — that is, what the subjects were eating before the study began, an important variable in studies relating to diet. (Twelve studies, by the way, constitutes a huge amount of research in the field of nutrition. Indeed, the fact that the researchers could find twelve randomized controlled trials, many of them of reasonably high quality, in just the previous decade indicates that this is one of the more-studied questions in nutrition science.)

Most of the studies that adequately controlled for what people were otherwise eating found that altering cholesterol consumption had little to no effect on blood LDL — the bad cholesterol. Small subgroups of participants with certain genes appeared to be more susceptible to higher blood cholesterol levels resulting from eating foods high in cholesterol, but even in those few subjects, the link wasn't as strong as many presumed.

Thus, we have relatively good data about the cholesterol question. Most of the studies indicate that there's no relationship between your intake of cholesterol and the amount of cholesterol in your body. Yet even with all of these data, I still get lectures from people (including my mother) telling me that this food or that food has too much cholesterol in it. I wonder what James Vaupel and John Graham would think of these doubters.

In 1980, these two researchers ran the numbers on eggs and cholesterol and found that the existing dietary recommendations made little sense. Back then, before many of the randomized controlled trials were done, and when most people were still convinced that eggs were the devil, these scientists estimated (with some pretty impressive math) that eliminating two dozen eggs from the diet of a very high-risk 48-year-old man might cut his chances of dying before age 60 by 0.5%. To put it another way, they calculated that eliminating 19,000 eggs from your diet over a lifetime might extend your life by twenty days — all at the end, of course, when you're not squeezing as much out of your days as you were when you were younger and subjecting yourself, day after day, to those revolting egg-white omelets.

It turns out that many of Vaupel and Graham's estimates were conservative. They depended on everyone being a responder to consumed cholesterol, but as we've seen, 70% of us are hyporesponders. So eliminating those eggs would likely do nothing at all for those folks.

Luckily, scientific consensus about dietary cholesterol is beginning to shift, and public opinion seems to be changing along with it. In December 2014, the USDA Dietary Guidelines Advisory Committee met to discuss possible changes to the guidelines for the United States. (As you may recall from chapter 1, this is the group of scientists that reviews all the evidence and makes recommendations to the government about what should be in the USDA Dietary Guidelines, which are put out every five years.) After the advisory committee's meeting, the committee published a report in which they acknowledged that "cholesterol is not considered a nutrient of concern for overconsumption." To the USDA's credit, when it released the updated guidelines in 2015, it used that same wording.

Americans can be forgiven for being surprised that their government was suddenly telling them not to worry about how much cholesterol they were eating. For decades, most of us had been watching our cholesterol intake religiously. So perhaps it also shouldn't come as any surprise that this new wisdom has been slow to catch on.

RAW EGGS ARE FINE, TOO

I've spent years trying to liberate my friends from their fears of eggs. I thought the new USDA guidelines would finally do the trick. But our collective fear of eggs' cholesterol content may have seeped into our subconscious — because even when I present the latest research to people, I find they've already invented other, equally spurious reasons to fear eggs.

For instance, lots of people seem to think that eggs are more likely to be dirty or infected than a whole host of other foods. As with many myths, this one has a kernel of truth, because eggs were once linked to a risk of infection from *Salmonella enteritidis*. If you wander over to the Centers for Disease Control and Prevention's website, you'll learn that you have to take "special care" to avoid getting salmonella when eating eggs. You need to keep them refrigerated at all times, avoid cracked or dirty eggs, and wash anything that might touch raw eggs, including "counter tops, utensils, dishes, and cutting boards," as well as, of course, your hands. The CDC further warns that even when eggs appear germ-free, their insides can contain salmonella, so you must cook them thoroughly before eating them.

That collective groan you hear is the millions of children who are being told they can't lick the bowl or the mixers when their parents make cookies or cakes. Sure, that's like the best part of baking — but you could get salmonella, so no cookie dough for you!

Please don't think I'm minimizing how terrible it is to get salmonella. It's not fun. And certain groups for whom salmonella can be especially dangerous — the elderly, infants, and immunocompromised people, to name a few — should all take special care. My point is simply that we need to understand the real risk of getting salmonella from eggs and make decisions based on that information — not our fears about some worst-case scenario. If we made every decision based on fear alone, we would never get in cars.*

Decades ago, the threat of contracting salmonella from eggs was a much bigger concern than it is today. In 1990, the USDA traced a salmonella outbreak back to some egg producers in the Northeast. In response, Pennsylvania egg producers, federal and state agriculture departments, Penn State, and the University of Pennsylvania took action to reduce egg contamination. The result was the Pennsylvania Egg Quality Assurance Program, which decreased the percentage of Pennsylvania poultry houses contaminated with salmonella from 38% in 1992 to 8% in 2010.

That percentage may still sound high. But in the bad old days of 1992, the risk of being exposed to salmonella was still pretty small, at 2.6 per 10,000 eggs. By 2010, it had dropped to about 1.2 per 10,000 eggs. Put another way, this means that in 2010, 0.012% of the eggs in the United States *might* have been contaminated with salmonella.

So the number of contaminated eggs out there is incredibly low. And keep in mind that not everyone who eats a contaminated egg will get sick. The human body is exceptionally good at fighting off disease. Moreover, even if you do get sick from eating an infected egg, odds are you will hardly even notice. Studies predict that 94% of people who contract salmonella will recover completely without any medical care at all. About

---

* This is one of the best examples of understanding risk. Cars are the number one killers of children outside of infancy. More kids die in accidents every year than from any other single cause. If we focused on that fact alone, we'd ban kids from getting in cars. But we also know that cars improve our lives in many ways, so we accept this real risk of death in order to get the benefits they provide. That's only rational. Likewise, we need to weigh the risks and the rewards when making decisions about what we eat, including eggs.

5% will visit a doctor, and 0.5% will be hospitalized. Only 0.05% will die, and most of those people will likely have some underlying medical condition.

Here's another way of thinking about the real risk of getting sick from contaminated eggs. If you live in the United States, and you accept that your risk of coming into contact with salmonella in any one egg is 0.012%, you could eat one raw egg every week (which would require making a lot of cookie batter) for one hundred years (which most of us couldn't, since we won't live that long) and still have a good chance of never eating an egg with salmonella. Even if you did encounter that egg, you most likely wouldn't get sick. And even if you did get sick, you most likely won't care.

With all of that said, it's good to make a habit of food safety. You should keep your eggs refrigerated, you should rinse them before cracking them, and you should wash everything that touches them with soap and water.

But also live a little. Enjoy raw cookie dough once in a while. The risk is so much lower than many others you run every day.

THE BOTTOM LINE

Eggs are safe to eat. Neither their cholesterol content nor the risk of contracting salmonella from them is a reason not to eat them, whether cooked or raw, especially if you're a healthy adult.

That doesn't mean that having high levels of bad cholesterol in your blood isn't dangerous. It also doesn't mean that people who are taking drugs to help reduce their cholesterol levels don't actually need them. But it does mean that eating eggs — or other high-cholesterol foods, for that matter — is not going to make much difference in your blood cholesterol levels if you are one of the roughly 70% of people who do not "respond" to dietary cholesterol.

So how do you know if you are a responder or a hyporesponder? Simply ask your doctor. Together, you can try to figure out whether changing the amount of cholesterol you consume will make a big difference in the amount of cholesterol in your blood. Chances are that you can stop worrying about how much dietary cholesterol you consume. For most people, it just doesn't make that much difference.

My daughter has always loved eggs. When she was little, my wife and I limited her consumption because we believed that the cholesterol in them was bad for her. No longer. She now eats eggs, as do my boys, as often as she likes. We also let them lick the bowl. As for me, I'm back to eating regular omelets — yolks and all.

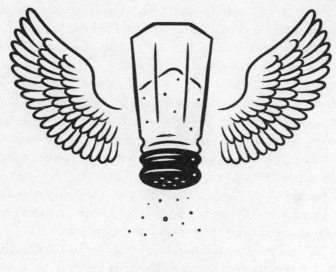

Four

SALT

I LOVE cooking shows. They're like catnip to me. And if I've learned one thing from watching these programs, especially the ones that are judged by a panel of hypercritical restaurateurs and chefs, it's that people seem to dislike food that hasn't been seasoned enough. Specifically, they seem to really have an aversion to food that doesn't have enough salt. When a judge on a cooking show utters those four fateful words — "This needs more seasoning"—it's safe to assume that the contestant has underutilized the saltcellar.

There's just something special about sodium chloride, the chemical compound that makes up salt. We need both sodium and chloride to live; these ions are critical to cell health and biochemistry. So it shouldn't be surprising that we crave them in our food.

Most of us enjoy the taste of salt, but its usefulness in the kitchen doesn't end there. Salt also suppresses the bitter taste in foods, which lets the other (better) tastes get through.* It tenderizes meat and can be used to dehydrate foods, concentrating other flavors. Research shows that it can even improve the "thickness" of foods, enhancing sweetness and rounding out other flavors. When you add salt to a soup, it doesn't just make the soup salty. It also makes it feel more substantial.

Infants are somewhat indifferent to salt, but by the time they reach six months, they begin to like it. It hasn't been proven, but there are people who theorize that as small children are exposed to salt, they want more and more of it. Since we put salt in pretty much everything these days, the logic goes, we build kids, and later adults, who want lots of it.

The fact is, however, that humans always craved salt, even when it was a scarce commodity. Throughout history, people have recognized salt as a basic necessity of life. Changes in their diets and the climates in which they lived made salt more essential for keeping the proper balance of water in our bodies. In hot, dry areas, consuming enough salt—with water, of course —was important for survival. Salt was also instrumental in the preservation of food before the invention of refrigeration. Meat soaked in salt water or packed in dry salt was much less likely

---

* Salt is one of the five basic tastes. The others are bitter, sweet, sour, and umami—the "earthy" taste you get from monosodium glutamate (MSG), the subject of chapter 10.

to spoil than the fresh stuff. This cured meat was an important source of food for many ancient (and some not-so-ancient) humans, sustaining our ancestors when times got tough.

It wasn't always easy for people to get their hands on salt. The word "salary" actually comes from "salt," and in the Roman Empire, salt was so rare that people used it as currency. Dating back to antiquity, Venice enjoyed a salt monopoly that made the city prosperous and helped it become a regional power. Salt was one of the reasons pioneers ventured west in America. Before the Revolutionary War, colonists relied on the British Empire to provide them with salt. After the war, they had to find their own supplies.

Some biologists point out that other animals don't have the need to salt their food. They will, though, often eagerly consume it when offered.

As I have already, and will again in later chapters, I caution you not to make too large an inference about human health from other animals. Most animals are day-to-day eaters, less picky than we are and much more likely to consume whatever food is available to them. Humans also aren't willing to dedicate as much time to getting food as most animals must.

Today, as with many things, we've made it too easy to get our hands on salt. And because of that, some people are consuming too much. But as with many of the other food items in this book, that doesn't mean you're necessarily eating more than your healthy share of it. In fact, some of you might not be getting enough.

SALT AND HIGH BLOOD PRESSURE

You've likely heard the claim that salt consumption can raise your blood pressure to unhealthy levels. This is an idea that dates back at least a century and is the source of most "salt is bad for you" reasoning. It's also not quite as clear-cut as that simple logic would lead you to believe. Salt consumption does seem to increase blood pressure — but that doesn't necessarily mean you should be consuming less.

Most experts believe that the first connection between salt consumption and high blood pressure was made in France in 1904. In a study conducted that year, two researchers followed six people with high blood pressure for three weeks. They put those people on three different diets, probably switching the subjects to a new diet every week. One regimen consisted of two liters of milk a day (and almost no salt). A second consisted of the milk plus protein, meat, and eggs (and still little salt). The third consisted of the milk plus two liters of broth (which contained a lot of salt).

The scientists who thought up these cruel and unusual meal plans also measured how much salt the patients excreted in their urine every day, using this measurement to deduce how much the subjects were eating. (It's much easier to measure people's intake of sodium by how much they excrete than how much they eat.) The researchers found that when people were consuming small amounts of salt, they were peeing out more than they were taking in; when they were eating lots of salt, however, they were taking in more than they were peeing out. What's more, when they were ingesting more salt, their blood pressure was higher.

I hope I've taught you enough about research to make you skeptical of any study that follows such a small sample of people for such a short amount of time. It's not even clear that this was a randomized or blinded trial, or that the scientists used reasonable criteria when picking people for inclusion in the study. They also did not clearly specify how they defined "high" levels of blood pressure.

This is not the kind of study you'd want to pay much attention to, let alone use to set policy about dietary health or make decisions about your diet. Yet, for the next few decades, some people in the medical profession began to treat high blood pressure by lowering salt. This trend only gained steam in the late 1940s, when a researcher named Walter Kempner demonstrated that a low-salt diet could be used to treat five hundred patients with high blood pressure. Never mind that this diet consisted of plain rice and fruit and was almost impossible to stick to. A lawsuit even alleged that Dr. Kempner actually resorted to physical punishment to make his subjects compliant with the diet.

This approach — treating blood pressure by lowering salt intake — didn't work out too well, for a variety of reasons. For one thing, when solutions that require lifestyle changes (such as switching to a bland diet of plain rice and fruit) seem too hard to maintain, we often try to find pharmaceutical solutions that will have the same effect. Salt balance is a perfect example. Drugs that cause us to increase our salt excretion — commonly known as diuretics — became more widely available in the mid-1950s and made it easier for doctors to alter their patients' salt balance without putting them on crazy, unrealistically restrictive diets. These drugs can have significant side effects, though, including electrolyte imbalances, weakness, and even heart arrhythmias.

Ironically, however, there is actually good evidence that salt intake can be bad for people with high blood pressure. A study published in the *New England Journal of Medicine* in 2014 — the Prospective Urban and Rural Epidemiology (PURE) Study — confirms this. Analyzing the sodium levels in the urine of more than 100,000 people in eighteen countries, researchers found that people who consumed more sodium had significantly higher blood pressure than those who did not. Another analysis performed by the same group, and published in the same issue of the journal, went even further. It found that people who consumed more than 7 grams of sodium per day had a significantly higher chance of death than people who consumed 3 to 6 grams per day. People consuming very high levels of sodium had higher rates of heart attack, heart failure, and stroke as well.

Health researchers find results like these time and time again, and the conclusions are inescapable: People eating too much salt should consume less, lest they develop cardiovascular problems. People with high blood pressure should definitely limit their sodium intake as much as possible.

But does this mean that we should *all* steer clear of salt? No.

Many of us may get too little salt. Americans, for instance, consume 3.4 grams of sodium per day on average.* This is on the low end of the "safe zone" of 3 to 6 grams delineated in the 2014 *New England Journal of Medicine* study. Eat much less than that, and your health might suffer, as I explain in the next section.

Of course, not everyone agrees on how much salt is "safe." The U.S. Food and Drug Administration thinks that 3 to 6 grams is not low enough. It recommends 2.3 grams per day. The World Health Organization says it should be 2.0 grams. The American Heart Association goes even further and recommends that we consume no more than 1.5 grams of sodium per day.

But there's no rationale for these numbers. In 2013, a committee at the Institute of Medicine assessed the evidence concerning sodium intake around the world. The committee agreed

---

* Because salt intake has a lower bound (zero) and no higher bound (people can consume *a lot*), more people consume less than 3.4 grams than consume more than 3.4 grams. Remember that when people say "Everyone is eating too much salt."

that efforts to reduce excessive sodium intake were warranted. But they cautioned that no evidence existed to recommend a very low-salt diet. They hoped that future research would inform the potential benefits of a diet in which sodium intake was 1.5 to 2.3 grams per day—the levels promoted by other groups.

The *New England Journal of Medicine* study did just that. In addition to tracking the health of people on high-sodium diets, it compared their health outcomes with those of people on very low-sodium diets. What the researchers found is concerning: Compared with those who consumed 3 to 6 grams of sodium per day, people who consumed less than 3 grams per day had an even higher risk of death or cardiovascular events than those who consumed more than 7 grams.

This result would be shocking if the medical community hadn't seen it before. But we have. In 2011, a study published in *JAMA*, the *Journal of the American Medical Association*, followed 3,681 people over almost a decade. These researchers, too, found that excessive salt intake was associated with high blood pressure. They also found that a low-sodium diet was associated with higher mortality from cardiovascular causes.

Apparently, having too much salt *or* too little can lead to a heart attack or stroke. So why do experts and organizations urge people to go from one extreme to the other? Sadly, we do this far too often in medicine—take findings about one group and apply them to everyone else.

WHO NEEDS SALT?

Like most other things in dietary health, salt intake is not a one-size-fits-all issue. A recent meta-analysis makes this point quite well. This study examined how salt intake is associated with cardiovascular events and death, but it added to the discussion by including hypertension, a fancy term for high blood pressure.

The researchers wanted to see how salt intake affected those outcomes for people with high blood pressure versus people with normal blood pressure. Distinguishing the effects of salt on these different groups would be important, because if the researchers could figure out whether — and how — salt affects people with high blood pressure differently than people with normal blood pressure, medical professionals would be able to tailor recommendations about salt intake to each group.

The meta-analysis reviewed data from four large studies that collectively compared more than 133,000 people from forty-nine countries. The researchers in these studies had followed their subjects for a median of more than four years, and the subjects themselves were about evenly split between people with and without hypertension.

The results revealed that salt did indeed affect people with high blood pressure and normal blood pressure differently. The researchers found that people with high blood pressure seemed to have more of a sensitivity to sodium. Subjects with hypertension experienced almost double the rise in blood pressure as people without hypertension when they consumed the same amount of salt (even though neither saw a huge increase). The researchers also found that people with high blood pressure who consumed more than 7 grams of sodium a day had significantly greater rates of cardiac events and death than those who consumed 4 to 5 grams. By contrast, people with normal blood pressure had no increased risk at the higher level of consumption.

In other words, consuming too much salt appears to be a risk factor for bad outcomes for people with hypertension. But that same concern isn't seen in people with normal blood pressure.

Surprisingly, the meta-analysis also showed that people with hypertension could harm themselves more by eating too little salt than by having too much. Those who consumed less than 3 grams of sodium per day had a higher risk of bad outcomes than those who consumed 4 to 5 grams, and even worse outcomes than people who consumed more than 7 grams.

This finding—that having too little salt is more dangerous than having too much—applies to people with normal blood pressure, too. Subjects with normal blood pressure who consumed less than 3 grams of salt per day had higher levels of risk than those consuming 4 to 5 grams. These results held even when the researchers excluded subjects with known cardiovascular disease.

This meta-analysis both reinforces and debunks the conventional wisdom about salt and cardiovascular health. It lends credence to the idea that people with high blood pressure who consume an excessive amount of salt should reduce their intake. But it also suggests that people with normal blood pressure can increase their salt intake without seeing much of a difference in their health.

Troublingly, the study's other big finding—that the push for very low levels of salt in our diets may be doing more harm than good—is supported by a growing body of evidence. Even more disturbingly, policy makers seem incapable of absorbing this nuance. The 2015 USDA Dietary Guidelines, for instance, continue to insist that Americans should be lowering their sodium intake, when the data seem to suggest that many of them might actually want to do the exact opposite.

THE SODIUM PARADOX

Whether you should be eating less salt or more, our food system makes it hard to strike the right balance when it comes to sodium intake. Perhaps the biggest problem with sodium these days isn't how much salt you're adding to your food from the shaker on your dining table; it's the amount of salt that's been put into the prepared foods you buy at the store and order in restaurants.

It's estimated that about 80% of the sodium Americans consume every day is from salt that's been added to food as it's been processed. For instance, a single slice of white bread can contain up to 230 mg of sodium. Three ounces of turkey breast from the deli can contain more than 1,000 mg. A slice of American cheese can contain more than 450 mg.

You probably don't even know the salt is there. It's in prepared pasta sauce, frozen pizza, canned soup, and more. The Center for Science in the Public Interest keeps a running tab of the amount of sodium in various foods sold throughout the United States. The Cheesecake Factory's Fried Chicken & Waffles Benedict contains 3,390 mg of sodium, which is what most people might eat all day. Dave & Buster's Short Rib & Cheesy Mac Stack has the exact same amount. But these are nothing compared with the Whole Hog Burger and sides at Uno Pizzeria & Grill. That meal contains a whopping 9,790 mg of sodium. Eat either of the first two dishes and almost anything else during the day, and it's likely you're going to be wandering into the "high" range of salt intake, where almost everyone agrees you're consuming too much. Eat just the Whole Hog Burger, and you're already there.

Let's face it — companies and restaurants use salt for the same reason cooking show contestants do: because it makes their food taste better. But that makes it very hard for people who want to monitor their salt consumption to do so. If you stopped eating out and stopped eating processed foods, you could probably cut your salt intake by a huge amount without even trying. Too few people seem to be able to accomplish this, however.

You can't just tell people to do it themselves. As a pediatrician, I've been listening for many years to complaints about how school lunches aren't healthy. Among other things, people complain that they are too high in sodium. Because of that, I've heard many calls for parents to be more active and to make lunches for their kids instead. But no one ever fights for parents to have more money or time to make those meals. As a result, when parents pack lunches for their kids, those lunches often have more sodium in them than the lunches provided by the school.*

Mindful of how much salt can end up in prepared foods, many activists are pushing the FDA to impose restrictions on how foods can be prepared, packaged, and labeled with respect to sodium. Their intent is good. Studies using blinded taste tests have shown that restaurants could reduce the amount of salt they put in foods without much damage to their bottom line. And many companies, mindful of the growing consumer movement for low-salt food options, have done just that. A number of the most prominent fast-food chains have cut the sodium in many of their offerings. They don't like to talk about it, though, because when people hear "healthier," they often think "less tasty."

Other companies have tried to placate the anti-sodium

---

* This is backed up by research. A study of eight elementary schools in Texas looked at the lunches kids were bringing in versus those provided in the cafeteria. It found that those made at home contained 1,110 mg of salt on average versus less than 640 mg of salt in the meals offered by the schools.

movement by changing the type of salt they provide. For instance, kosher salt actually has less sodium per volume than table salt, and some restaurants have started to offer that in the hope that people will use similar amounts and get less sodium. Of course, kosher salt tastes less "salty" per volume, too, so there's a chance diners will just use more of it to get the same effect — not a perfect solution, by any means.

When policy makers get involved in the salt wars, their interventions tend to be similarly misguided. In New York City, for instance, the city government passed regulations that required chain restaurants to add warnings to their menus about items that contain 2,300 mg of sodium or more. But that's a *huge* amount of sodium: it's actually the FDA limit for daily consumption. Something with that much sodium in it would be really salty; if you don't already know it's a very high-sodium food just by its taste, you likely aren't paying attention. And anyway, the underlying problem isn't that some foods have a ton of salt in them; it's that companies are sneaking sodium into foods that we don't even think have much.

Sodium levels in prepared foods probably won't go down across the board unless the government makes some major changes in regulations, which many Americans seem reluctant to allow. But keep in mind that we're talking about *prepared foods* here, not all foods. If you're eating enough processed foods or restaurant fare for the sodium content to have a significant impact on your health, odds are you're hurting yourself by overconsuming other ingredients as well.

THE BOTTOM LINE

While more than 95% of people in eighteen countries consume more than 3 grams of sodium per day, only 22% consume more than 6 grams. For healthy people, the amount they are already consuming is likely okay. As far as these folks are concerned, the very low-sodium goals pushed by many health organizations are not only difficult to achieve but probably not advisable from a medical standpoint either. Remember that such diets are associated with a higher risk of cardiac events and even death.

To be sure, we need more information about how low salt intake affects our health. Large randomized controlled trials are needed to assess the value of very low-sodium diets. Usually such prospective trials are meant to confirm the associations we see in cohort or case-control studies. In this case, however, the epidemiologic studies suggest that very low-sodium diets may be harmful, not beneficial.

According to the FDA, about one-third of adults have high blood pressure, and they may want to reduce their salt intake. For the rest of us, the dire warnings about sodium we get from the health establishment might not apply.

With salt, as with so many other things, we have to be careful not to overdo or underdo it. Too many calories are bad for us. That doesn't mean we should consume none. Too little exercise can be unhealthy. That doesn't mean we should work out to the point of hurting ourselves. Too much sun can cause cancer. That doesn't mean we should never go outside.

It's a cliché, but it's true: moderation in everything. Processed foods often contain more sodium than we need or want, and we're usually better off cooking for ourselves. But if the dish you make at home tastes like it needs more salt, it probably does.

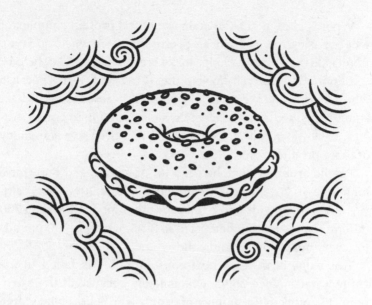

GLUTEN

MANY people today fear and loathe gluten. Fewer of us actually know what it is.

I'm amazed at how many products are marketed as "gluten-free." Candy is labeled gluten-free, as is soda, meat, and even vegetables. What's odd is that none of these foods have ever contained gluten. The companies pronouncing them gluten-free are just trying to trick you into thinking they're somehow healthier now.

What is gluten? It's the main structural protein complex of wheat, barley, rye, and triticale (a cross between wheat and rye). It's elastic in nature and helps make bread chewy and delicious.

Eliminating gluten from your diet is not easy. That's because wheat, barley, and rye are in all kinds of processed foods. Wheat is in breads, soups, pasta, cereals, sauces, and many other edibles. Barley is in food coloring, malts, and beer. Rye is in many of those products, too.

People around the globe eat a lot of gluten, and have for a long time. In 2014, wheat accounted for about 20% of the calories eaten worldwide, more than any other food. More than 700 million tons of it were harvested in 2013, which is 200 pounds for every man, woman, and child.

Ironically, however, wheat consumption has fallen in the United States since 2000. This is likely because of the astronomical uptick in the number of people who believe that gluten causes health problems.

Our reduced consumption, however, clearly hasn't reduced the incidence of gluten "problems." This is because gluten is perfectly fine for the vast majority of people. Not everyone can eat it, of course. If you have celiac disease or a wheat allergy, avoiding gluten is pretty much a must. But if you are "gluten sensitive," you aren't necessarily in the same boat.

WHEAT ALLERGY AND CELIAC DISEASE

There are three groups of people for whom avoiding gluten may be necessary: those with a wheat allergy, celiac disease, or gluten sensitivity. These conditions are not the same thing, however, and the first two are much more clear-cut than the third.

People with a wheat allergy, as you might imagine, need to avoid wheat, and they can do so by going gluten-free.

Wheat allergy is pretty rare. In Europe, the prevalence is 0.1%, which makes it less common than allergies to cow's milk, eggs, soy, peanuts, tree nuts, fish, and shellfish. In Asia, the prevalence is between 0.08% and 0.21%. In the United States, it's somewhere between 0.4% and 1%. Children account for a good proportion of those percentages, and many of them eventually outgrow the allergy.

Many people believe that we have become too inclusive in what's defined as an actual allergy, but if you've been diagnosed by a doctor as having a wheat allergy, you probably need to consume a wholly or mostly wheat-free diet (depending on the severity of the allergy). You might even be cautioned to avoid gluten in addition to wheat. That may be overkill, though. Just because you need to avoid wheat doesn't mean you need to avoid gluten in all its forms — or necessarily should. Wheat-free diets can be much more permissive than gluten-free diets, and thus are easier to maintain and less likely to leave you deficient in some nutrient.

If you have celiac disease, however, that means you basically have an immune reaction to gluten. Celiac patients should absolutely avoid gluten altogether.

First noted about 130 years ago, celiac disease was described in patients who seemed malnourished and had especially smelly, pale stools. Initially, physicians didn't know what caused celiac disease, but they had a hunch that altering patients' diets might be the solution. At first, they tried instructing celiac patients to avoid milk, fruits, and vegetables, but none of these dietary changes seemed to have any effect on their underlying condition. Later, physicians thought a low-fat diet might be the cure, but that didn't work too well either.

By the 1940s, celiac researchers had finally set their sights on wheat, thanks in part to the deprivations of World War II. During the war, embargoes and famines left many people in

Europe without bread and other wheat-based products. Ironically, celiac patients saw their gut health improve remarkably under these otherwise dire circumstances. After the war, with this clue in hand, scientists were able to identify gluten as the cause of celiac disease.

If you have celiac disease, when any food with gluten in it hits your small intestine, something makes your body go a little nuts. Your immune system becomes convinced there's a problem to fix and shifts into high gear. But with nothing truly dangerous to battle, your body's defense system winds up doing more harm than good. Over time, the lining of your small intestine gets chronically inflamed, and you can't absorb all of the nutrients you need. This can cause weight loss, bloating, and diarrhea; it can also lead to other parts of the body being denied the nutrition they need.

One of the challenges of celiac disease is that most people don't have any noticeable symptoms, making the condition very difficult to diagnose. About 20% of people with the disease have constipation, and 10% are obese. As many as 75% of kids with celiac disease are overweight or obese. They don't look malnourished, however, as you might expect of children whose bodies are being starved of nutrients.

Doctors can rely on at least a few celiac facts when attempting to diagnose it. For instance, some people are more likely to have the disease than others. It runs in families, so if your relatives have celiac disease, you're at a higher risk for it. Celiac disease is also more common in people with type 1 diabetes, Down syndrome, and Turner syndrome. It can be more common in those with autoimmune thyroid disease or microscopic colitis as well.

Certain blood tests can help doctors determine if someone has celiac disease, but the real gold standard for detection is endoscopy, in which a doctor inserts a camera and a tube into the patient's throat in order to look at the small intestine. The doctor also will take a biopsy.

For people who are diagnosed with celiac disease, the only real treatment is a gluten-free diet. There is no cure. Patients usually start to feel better pretty fast once they stop consuming gluten, but complete healing of the small intestine can take years. Furthermore, if they start eating gluten again, all of their problems will likely recur.

A recent study estimated that the prevalence of celiac disease in the United States is 0.71%, meaning that about 1 in 141 people have it. That's similar to the rate in many European countries. Unfortunately, most cases go undiagnosed, which is one of the reasons people have latched onto the theory that celiac disease and therefore gluten are the causes of so many dietary problems around the world. We know the disease is there, but too few people realize they have it.

I'm immensely sympathetic to the problem of celiac disease. Given the statistics I just mentioned, about 3 million Americans are likely to suffer from it, many of whom go undiagnosed. That is, to some extent, the fault of doctors like myself. A study published in the *Journal of General Internal Medicine* surveyed more than 2,400 patients with celiac disease. Only 11% had been diagnosed by their primary care providers; the rest had been diagnosed by someone else — usually a medical specialist whom they had to seek out because their primary care providers couldn't help. The researchers who conducted this study also surveyed primary care physicians and found that only 35% of them had ever diagnosed celiac disease. That's not a very good track record, considering that doctors are statistically likely to have at least a few patients with the disorder.

Research has also shown that doctors will often misdiagnose

celiac disease as another condition. People diagnosed with irritable bowel syndrome are four times as likely to have celiac disease as people without IBS, meaning we often mistake IBS for celiac. Patients diagnosed and treated for iron and folate deficiencies sometimes turn out to have celiac disease. There's even one case report of a child who was diagnosed with autism but turned out to have celiac disease.

When the medical system fails people as widely as it has with celiac disease, patients start self-diagnosing. If your stomach feels lousy, you might wonder if you have the disease and put yourself on a gluten-free diet. If you end up feeling better, you may become convinced that gluten was the source of your misery, when really something else may have been bothering you — or when your improvement was the result of the placebo effect, rather than from a reduction of intestinal inflammation. If you think you have celiac disease, you need to see a doctor. Only a physician can make the diagnosis.

Because we believe that most people with celiac disease go undiagnosed, some patient advocates have argued that we should screen everyone for the disease. However, the U.S. Preventive Services Task Force, which makes recommendations for medical screening, has found that there isn't good evidence to support widespread screening, even among populations that are at increased risk. Biopsies aren't necessarily without their own risks, and celiac disease isn't common enough to warrant universal action. As a result, doctors still reserve testing for patients who have symptoms consistent with the illness.

Celiac disease is serious, and I don't want anyone reading this to think that I'm minimizing it in any way. If you have celiac disease, you absolutely need a gluten-free diet. But that may not be true for people with the other conditions discussed in the remainder of this chapter.

PEOPLE WITH GLUTEN SENSITIVITY MIGHT NEED
TO AVOID GLUTEN — MAYBE

The number of people who suffer from celiac disease and wheat allergy is relatively small. Other folks claim to have "gluten intolerance" or "gluten sensitivity," which is not an autoimmune problem (like celiac disease) or an allergic problem (like wheat allergy). It's something different, with a range of symptoms that have been attributed to gluten.

It's not as if people who claim to be gluten sensitive have no reason to do so. In a study published in the *American Journal of Gastroenterology* in 2011, researchers randomized thirty-four patients who said they were gluten sensitive to receive one of two interventions. All were put on a gluten-free diet. But half of them were also given a gluten-free muffin and two slices of gluten-free bread each day. The other half were given a muffin and bread containing gluten. Although more people in the second group complained of worsening symptoms (pain, bloating, tiredness, and decreased satisfaction with their stool consistency), 40% of those in the first, totally gluten-free group also complained of such symptoms. The researchers concluded, "'Non-celiac gluten intolerance' may exist, but no clues to the mechanism were elucidated."

This brief, ambiguous statement set off a firestorm. People started blaming gluten for a variety of things they found wrong with their lives or health. Books capitalizing on the hysteria were published. One, David Perlmutter's *Grain Brain,* declared that gluten "represents one of the greatest and most under-recognized health threats to humanity."

Let's remember, humans have been consuming gluten for thousands of years and have managed to take over the planet quite effectively in spite of that. Some people have argued that modern wheat has more gluten in it than the wheat consumed long ago, but scientists have looked into this and found that — at least in the United States in the twentieth and twenty-first centuries — wheat breeding has not led to an increase in the protein content or gluten content of wheat. So it doesn't seem as though the gluten our ancestors were consuming was somehow better for them than the gluten we ingest today.

Nor has the consumption of wheat flour been steadily rising in recent decades. The annual intake of wheat flour peaked at about 225 pounds per person in 1880, thereafter declining to a low of 110 pounds in the early 1970s. It then started to rise again, reaching 146 pounds by 2000, nowhere near the amount of wheat flour — and therefore gluten — Americans were eating in 1880. It seems unlikely, therefore, that gluten is a greater problem today than it was in the past simply because we're consuming more of it.

Millions of people, however, are unaware of, or unimpressed by, these findings. In 2014, it was estimated that Americans would spend more than $15 billion on gluten-free products in 2016. Gluten-free has become not only a huge fad but also a huge business. Even many of my friends — who are normally better informed about this stuff than most people — have started buying into the idea that gluten is horrible.

Remember that much of this began with a small study of thirty-four people. The results were not a slam dunk in terms of convincing people that those giving up gluten will see absolute improvements. In fact, lots of people argued against the findings.

Rather than rest on their laurels, these researchers continued to study gluten sensitivity specifically. They set up a better study to confirm their findings. This time they used a much more sophisticated design, involving people consuming varying levels of gluten over the course of the study to see how their symptoms changed. Their findings this time? "We found no evidence of specific or dose-dependent effects of gluten in patients with non-celiac gluten sensitivity placed diets." In other words, the gluten-free diet made no difference in relation to gluten sensitivity.

The researchers went even further in attempting to rein in the monster they had helped create. In a study published in 2014, they examined people who claimed to have gluten sensitivity. Of the 147 patients they studied, 72% didn't meet the established criteria for that diagnosis, despite having made the self-diagnosis or been given it, most often by a non-physician. Further, in 25% of these people, symptoms were poorly controlled even with a gluten-free diet.

As with many other areas of pseudoscience, when one idea fails, people soon latch onto another. When the evidence against gluten became weaker, scientists began to turn their attention to fermentable oligo-, di-, monosaccharides and polyols, otherwise known as FODMAPs. FODMAPs are present in gluten-containing foods, but they also can be found in foods that contain no gluten, such as onions, avocados, and garlic. Clearly, this casts an even wider net and gives some people a whole new list of foods to avoid. Unfortunately, the efficacy of these diets, and the means by which we can diagnose the people who might benefit from them, are just as unproven as the concept of gluten sensitivity itself.

AVOIDING GLUTEN MIGHT ACTUALLY HURT YOU

People have begun to blame all kinds of problems on gluten. These include things that have nothing to do with the intestines. Actress Jenny McCarthy, famous for her anti-vaccine advocacy, believes that a gluten- and casein-free diet was instrumental in improving the autism-like symptoms of her son. Elisabeth Hasselbeck, who used to cohost *The View* and actually has celiac disease, has promoted the diet as a great thing for most people, even those without the disorder. Actress Gwyneth Paltrow, never one to miss a food fad, also has advocated for a gluten-free diet as a means to improve one's health. Others swear that eliminating gluten from their diets improved the symptoms of diabetes, eczema, ADHD, Alzheimer's, and more. It shouldn't shock you that most of these claims are unsubstantiated by good research.

I'm not opposed to people eating more healthily. If you're avoiding gluten because it leads you to eat fewer processed foods, that's fine. If you do it to eat fewer carbs and more protein and vegetables, that's fine, too. Many people have found that when they give up gluten, they lose weight, although that probably has nothing to do with gluten. It's much more likely to be because when we give up gluten, we also give up bread, beer, refined carbohydrates, pasta, and many other processed foods that make us fat.

What's more, even if you think of gluten-free eating as a kind of weight-loss diet, there's no good evidence that it works better than any other mass-market diet. There's also no credible evidence that supports the idea that gluten is responsible for the obesity epidemic we're seeing worldwide, so there's not much logic in this sort of reasoning to begin with.

If anything, eating a gluten-free diet could cause you to gain weight, not lose it. A study published in 2006 followed 371 people with celiac disease who were put on a gluten-free diet. After two years, 81% of them gained weight. A similar study involving children found that after the kids switched to a gluten-free diet, the percentage who were overweight almost doubled. A study looking at the gluten-free diets of fifty-eight people with celiac disease in Spain found that those diets contained more fat and less fiber than the diets of people who ate gluten. More fat in your diet doesn't necessarily mean you're eating unhealthily (for more on this, see chapter 1), but it does mean that you're at greater risk of consuming too much.

Some good, though, has come out of our collective fixation on gluten. When I talk to people with celiac disease, they are often grateful that so many restaurants and food companies now offer so many gluten-free options. Not that long ago, they had very few choices available to them, and it was much harder to stick to a gluten-free diet. Now, many of their favorite foods are available in gluten-free varieties. For these people, life has improved quite a bit.

Don't forget, however, that people with celiac disease have no choice; they have to avoid gluten. For the rest of us, substituting gluten-free products for similar gluten-containing ones can backfire, big-time.

An article in the *Wall Street Journal* showed that gluten-free products sometimes are higher in carbs and sodium, and lower in fiber and protein, than similar gluten-containing products. Gluten-free cereals can have significantly fewer vitamins and minerals than those that contain gluten. Gluten-free flour substitutes such as rice starch, potato starch, and cornstarch are refined carbohydrates and can contribute to an unhealthy diet. A study following thousands of health professionals for more than twenty-five years found that those who ate less gluten consumed fewer whole grains (and received no protection from heart disease). Compared with regular bagels, gluten-free ones can have a quarter more calories, two and a half times the fat, half the fiber, and twice the sugar. They also cost way more.

Gluten-free diets can lead to deficiencies in nutrients such as vitamin B, folate, and iron. People on a strict gluten-free regimen also consume less magnesium, iron, and zinc. At the very least, those who have to eat gluten-free need education and help to counteract the inherent deficiencies that avoiding gluten can entail.

So why do so many people think they have a problem with gluten? The simplest explanation is that they are experiencing a *nocebo effect*. We've already discussed the placebo effect — when you experience a beneficial effect because you expect one to happen. A nocebo effect is the opposite. It's when you experience a *negative* effect for the same reason. In 2014, for instance, researchers published a meta-analysis of studies that looked at the nocebo effect with respect to pain. They found ten studies that involved giving people an inert substance and then suggesting that symptoms might worsen. When physicians did this, people reported significantly more pain than when the physicians didn't make any suggestions at all.

The take-home message here is that doctors should be careful what they say to patients, because suggesting that bad things might happen could actually make them happen. Given that we can't seem to turn around these days without being inundated with warnings about how bad gluten is for us, whether they come from friends, family, celebrities, or even the medical community, it's no surprise that people think they don't feel great when they consume it.

Another possible reason that gluten-free eating has gone mainstream is that it's riding the wave of an ongoing carbohydrate backlash. The Atkins diet, Paleo Diet, and so-called lifestyle plans like Whole30 are fundamentally low-carb eating programs that tell people to turn to protein and fats for more of their calories. Gluten, and its associated diseases and conditions, give people something to point to as evidence for why carbohydrates are unhealthy. It's not enough to acknowledge that carbs cause weight gain and obesity when we eat too much of them. It's easier to believe that they are actually bad for us on a chemical level.

This myth isn't losing its power, either. In a 2016 study, researchers used longitudinal survey data to estimate how many people in the United States underwent laboratory testing for celiac disease. They also looked at how many of the people surveyed had a prior diagnosis of celiac disease by a physician and were "adherent to" a gluten-free diet. They found that 106 of those who met these criteria were confirmed via laboratory testing to have celiac disease. The remaining 213 — over twice as many — did not. These may sound like small numbers, but they represent 1.76 million and 2.7 million people, respectively.

From 2009 to 2014, the prevalence of celiac disease was stable, but the prevalence of strict gluten-free diets was not. It went from 0.52% in 2009–2010 to 0.99% in 2011–2012 to 1.69% in 2013–2014. And this is undoubtedly an underestimate. Many people who go gluten-free are doing it without being entirely "adherent to" a gluten-free diet, and many others go out of their way simply to avoid gluten for reasons that don't seem to have much grounding, if any, in science.

THE BOTTOM LINE

If you have celiac disease, you need to be on a gluten-free diet. If you have a proven wheat allergy, you need to avoid wheat. But if you think you have gluten sensitivity? You'd probably be better off putting your energy and your dollars toward a different diet. Simply put, most people who think they have gluten sensitivity just don't.

It's impossible for me to prove that gluten sensitivity doesn't exist. It probably does. I imagine there are people who don't react well to gluten in ways that don't meet the definition of either celiac disease or wheat allergy. But it is likely pretty darn rare. Even proponents of non-celiac gluten sensitivity have said that the prevalence varies in different populations from as low as 0.63% to as much as 6%. Whatever the actual percentage, it is nowhere near the one-third of consumers who are trying to shun gluten-containing products.

While there's almost no evidence that a gluten-free diet will do these consumers any good at all, it does make food companies quite a bit of money. Sales of products with gluten-free labels have gone from $11.5 billion worldwide in 2010 to $23 billion in 2014. Companies even sold $2.1 billion of gluten-free dog food last year. Let me say that again: *gluten-free dog food.*

As with any other substance, if you think you have a sensitivity to gluten, it's best to discuss this with your physician. If he or she recommends a gluten-free diet, ask for the evidence behind the recommendation. I bet there won't really be any.

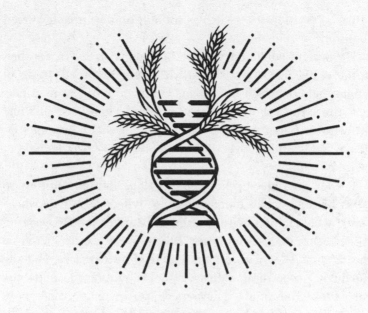

Six

GMOs

I N 1966 and 1967, India suffered back-to-back droughts. The resulting loss of crops led many observers to believe that the country was doomed to famine on a monstrous scale. This fear only became more acute when, in 1968, Stanford University professor Paul Ehrlich published his best-selling book, *The Population Bomb*. In it, Ehrlich predicted that in the 1970s and '80s, hundreds of millions of people would starve to death because certain countries, such as India, would be unable to feed themselves.

He clearly hadn't met Norman Borlaug. Two decades earlier, in the 1940s, Borlaug was in Mexico trying to breed strains of wheat that could fight off fungus and yield more grain at harvest time. He was massively successful. There was just one problem: so much grain grew on each stalk that it became top-heavy and would tip over. Plants that weren't upright couldn't be easily harvested.

Rather than give up his yield, Borlaug figured out how to cross his high-yield, fungus-resistant wheat with a Japanese dwarf wheat to produce a shorter, heavier variety. He was successful. Borlaug's "semidwarf" wheat significantly increased the amount of wheat farmers could grow per acre, and the Mexican agricultural industry quickly embraced it. By the early 1960s, the country's farmers were growing six times more wheat than they had been before the modified wheat was available.

In the mid- to late 1960s, as famine loomed over India and Ehrlich's book was hitting the shelves, Borlaug was working tirelessly to introduce his wheat into South Asia. The effects were miraculous. Soon after he brought his wheat to India, for instance, yields doubled. Famine was averted. Millions of lives were saved.

For his efforts, Borlaug won the Nobel Peace Prize in 1970. But his story did not end there.

Borlaug's semidwarf wheat ran into some problems that couldn't be fixed through simple crossbreeding. In Asia, the crop's water requirements seemed unsustainable in the long run. In Africa, farmers had a hard time finding enough fertilizer for the semidwarf wheat and protecting it from newer and stronger strains of fungus. The old methods didn't seem powerful enough.

So Borlaug began to support genetic modification. He noted that his earlier technique of crossbreeding crops was, at its root, a way of modifying their genes to improve human welfare. As science advanced, he reasoned, so did the means by which we could improve our crops, and thus our food supply.

Geneticists at the time were refining their techniques for re-engineering the code of life inside plant and animal cells, and they were all too happy to advance the cause Borlaug had championed. After all, he was the Nobel Prize–winning pioneer of what had come to be known as the green revolution. Surely this new effort, too, would be a boon to society.

But Borlaug's advocacy for genetically modified organisms — what we commonly refer to today as GMOs — would lead to an enormous backlash. Indeed, public antipathy toward GMOs would become so great that five years after his death in 2009, the respected British newspaper the *Guardian* could publish a blog post with the headline musing, "Norman Borlaug: Humanitarian Hero or Menace to Society?"

To understand how this could be — how an entire class of agricultural commodities could be so maligned, and how the savior of India could be tarred with the same brush — we need to understand what, exactly, GMOs are. But we also need to take a close look at the research about how they affect our health. Because while Borlaug's semidwarf wheat saved millions of lives, there are reasons to think that GMOs have saved even more. And there's not a shred of evidence to suggest that they have caused any harm.

A BRIEF HISTORY OF GMOs

Perhaps no food can divide people as quickly or as decisively as GMOs. Many people I know are convinced that these specially engineered fruits, vegetables, and animals are the grocery-story equivalent of Frankenstein's monster. Many groups, such as the Non-GMO Project and the Center for Food Safety, seem sure that GMOs are going to kill us all — and that if you don't agree with them, you're clearly a tool of Big Agriculture.

But as Borlaug's story shows us, we've been trying to alter the genes of the foods we eat for a long time. Since prehistory, farmers have bred livestock to increase their hardiness and size. They have also cross-pollinated and grafted different plants and trees to get newer, tastier, and all-around-better fruits and vegetables. In the 1930s, growers began subjecting seeds to radiation in the hope of causing desirable mutations. Today, scientists have the ability to change DNA with astonishing precision, using a revolutionary new gene-editing tool called CRISPR-Cas9.

To see why someone would want to rewrite the contents of a plant's or animal's genome, imagine that you're a farmer whose corn crop is being strangled by weeds. You've got a great weed killer, but it also kills the corn. What you really need is a weed killer that won't hurt the corn — or corn that won't be hurt by the weed killer.

Suppose that scientists have discovered bacteria that are immune to the weed killer. These bacteria are able to manufacture an enzyme that breaks down the poison in the herbicide before it can do any harm to the tiny organisms. You tell the scientists that you want your corn to develop the same ability, so they figure out which gene allows the bacteria to create the enzyme that makes it immune to the weed killer, then they go into the bacteria's DNA, snip out that gene, and place it in the DNA of some corn seeds. The corn plant that grows out of those seeds will be able to make the enzyme, and it, too, will be resistant to the weed killer. Problem solved.

This sounds like science fiction, but scientists have been able to do it for some time. If you — the farmer in this scenario — plant the GMO corn in your fields, you can spray them with the weed killer and be sure that everything will die but the corn itself. Using the same technology, scientists can also, theoretically, make crops that are more nutritious, able to grow in different climates, require less water and fertilizer, or are naturally resistant to certain diseases.

There's a lot of potential for good in GMO crops. It's also important to recognize that this kind of modification also occurs in nature. DNA mutations eventually confer adaptive benefits on certain species, allowing them to overcome such challenges without human intervention. This is Darwin's theory of evolution by natural selection at work. Genetic engineering just dramatically speeds up the process and allows for more specific changes than nature usually stumbles upon through the halting process of random mutation.

GMOs are also really common. More than 90% of the soybeans planted in the United States are GMOs. About 80% of the corn and cotton are, too. Well over half of the processed foods that you buy every day have some GMO in them. Most of the GMO crops worldwide are grown in Canada. Second place goes to Brazil, then Argentina, the United States, and India. In 2013, about 12% of all farmland in the world was growing GMOs.

Despite GMOs' ubiquity and their clear environmental and humanitarian benefits, many people are vehemently opposed to them. Their reasons vary widely, but one constant refrain is that GMOs are unhealthy because they are "unnatural," and therefore unsafe. But as I hope you'll agree by the time you've finished reading this chapter, that sort of reasoning is not just unscientific — it is wrong on a number of different levels.

THE CASES FOR AND AGAINST —
BUT MOSTLY FOR — GMOs

To date, there is no good evidence that GMO crops are any more dangerous to eat than non-GMO crops. But don't take my word for it.

In 2004, the Institute of Medicine and the National Research Council of the National Academy of Sciences put out a report reviewing all the available evidence about GMOs and health. They concluded that there was no evidence at all that GMOs posed any greater danger to people than conventionally grown foods.

The European Union conducted its own research into the safety of GMOs. According to its report, "The main conclusion to be drawn from the efforts of more than 130 research projects, covering a period of more than 25 years of research and involving more than 500 independent research groups, is that *biotechnology, and in particular GMOs, are not per se more risky than e.g. conventional plant breeding technologies*" (emphasis mine).

Health-wise and otherwise, GMOs are no better or worse than any other foods. The American Medical Association agrees. So does the National Academy of Sciences, Britain's Royal Society, and the World Health Organization. None of these organizations say that GMOs are completely safe. Rather, they say that GMOs are just as safe as conventionally grown foods. That's because even foods that don't contain GMOs aren't perfectly safe. Some people are allergic to certain foods. Others have bad reactions to foods for different reasons — for instance, people with celiac disease can't eat gluten without getting sick.

If GMOs aren't any more or less safe than other foods, that

means someone, somewhere, might have a bad reaction to them. But the risk is no greater or less than it is for any other foods.

That well-established fact doesn't seem to make GMO objectors feel safe, however. And if you're reading this in the United States, odds are you're in this camp. A Pew poll in 2015 asked Americans whether they thought it was generally safe or unsafe to eat GMOs. More than half said it was unsafe. Only about a third of the people said they thought GMOs were generally safe.

The same poll asked scientists from the American Association for the Advancement of Science, or AAAS, the same question. Ironically, only 11% of them thought GMOs were unsafe, whereas 88% said they were generally safe.

But most Americans, at least according to this poll, don't seem to care what scientists think. When they were asked whether they thought scientists had a clear understanding of the health effects of GMOs, two-thirds of the respondents said they didn't. In fact, Americans disagree with scientists on this issue more than just about any other, including a host of contentious topics such as vaccines, evolution, and even global warming.

Americans aren't the only ones panicked about GMOs. In Europe, regulations regarding their use and how they are sold are even stricter than in the United States. Many Asian countries refuse to buy any products that contain GMOs even in small quantities, and public concerns about their safety are even more widespread there than in the United States.

Why do people distrust science so much when it comes to GMOs? One reason is that they're worried about new allergies to these foods. Although companies usually test for allergies, critics think they could be doing more.

I don't disagree. But some people take this contention a step further and argue that since it's impossible to test for all allergies to GMO foods, consumers should be wary of all GMOs. That seems like a huge stretch. After all, we don't test non-GMO foods for all allergies, but that doesn't mean we should stop eating all those foods.

Another argument against GMO crops is that they lead to increased use of herbicides, which could be toxic. That possibility is worth studying, but it certainly hasn't been proven. And as I mentioned earlier, GMOs could actually *reduce* farmers' use of chemicals if the crops were engineered for that.

This objection to GMOs is connected to a larger one, which is that GMOs are bad for the environment. The evidence is mixed here, too. On the one hand, as I just mentioned, GMOs can, in many ways, lead to fewer chemicals being used. On the other hand, if farmers use more powerful chemicals, knowing that these won't kill their crops, this can lead to the development of resistant strains of pests. Moreover, it's possible that the genes we insert into crops can get out of the lab. This happened in Oregon in 2013. After a farmer there had sprayed some fields with the weed killer glyphosate, he noticed that some patches of wheat continued to grow. When he sent some samples to a lab, they were found to be a variety that Monsanto had developed, but discontinued before getting EPA approval, almost a decade earlier. No one knows how the wheat got into his fields.

Of course, non-GMO crops can gain these abilities as well. Bacteria can develop a resistance to antibiotics without any genetic modification on our part. Weeds can become resistant to herbicides without our tinkering with them. Life evolves.

An added complication in this debate is that much of the research on GMOs is being done by companies that have an inherent conflict of interest. GENera, the Genetic Engineering Risk Atlas, which gathers all the evidence it can on GMOs, has collected more than 1,080 studies that have looked at their relative risks. In general, only about a third of the studies — no small amount, but by no means the majority — were conducted by neutral third parties without any financial interest in the results.

In 2014, GENera published a systematic review of the independent research about GMOs. It looked at a decade's worth of the latest studies to describe the independent scientific consensus as of that time. The authors concluded, "The scientific research conducted so far has not detected any significant hazards directly connected with the use of GE [genetically engineered] crops; however, the debate is still intense."

An understatement, if there ever was one.

LABELING GMOs ISN'T NEARLY
AS HELPFUL AS IT SEEMS

Despite the evidence that GMOs are as safe as anything else we eat, many people want GMOs out of our foods. And if governments won't ban GMO crops (as they show no interest in doing), they want restaurants and food companies to at least stop using GMOs in the foods they serve and make.

Doing so would have consequences. Forcing companies to eliminate GMOs from their supply chains would cost consumers money, as the companies might have to bypass cheaper suppliers and pass the extra costs on to us. It would also lead people to believe that non-GMO foods are somehow better, even though there is no evidence to support that belief.

Eliminating GMOs wouldn't be easy. Chipotle learned that the hard way in 2015, when it declared that it would serve only GMO-free foods in its restaurants. It was then shown that the drinks in Chipotle's soda machines contained corn syrup that was genetically modified. Additionally, some of the meat the company used was from animals that had eaten GMO feed.

As Chipotle discovered, getting GMOs completely out of our food supply would be really hard. This is due in part to the fact that we can't easily define what is and what is not a GMO. Advocacy organizations, at least those that are actively focused on crops, don't seem to have a problem with the idea of cross-breeding plants naturally to produce desirable traits. But they do have a problem with transgenesis, the process of moving genes between species. (This is what I described earlier in my example of transferring DNA from bacteria to corn.) Most definitions of GMOs focus on this process: the incorporation of foreign DNA into an organism's genome.

But what if we just go into a plant and change its genes directly? Would the resulting organism still be a GMO? CRISPR-Cas9, the revolutionary gene-editing technology, has enormous potential for changing the genetic makeup of plants, and the fact that it involves genetic manipulation makes some people uncomfortable. Yet the U.S. government does not consider the affected plants to be GMOs.

How about the long-standing practice of irradiating seeds to cause mutations? This was tolerated long before the advent of GMOs. Ironically, it's much less controlled than other methods of genetic manipulation, and is much more likely to lead to unintended consequences, because it is much less precise. It, too, produces crops that aren't technically GMOs.

If we widen the definition of a GMO to include any organism created by human intervention, the term begins to look much less scary. Breeding animals or plants in an attempt to enhance certain features would fall under this definition. So would grafting trees. These processes are clearly safe; we've been doing them for millennia. They're also powerful tools in the fight to feed humanity. Who could argue that the world would be better off if Borlaug hadn't created semidwarf wheat, and millions of people had simply starved to death?

Bizarrely, people seem to have little concern about these same genetic techniques being used in medicine. Insulin, which has saved millions of people with diabetes, was originally produced using pancreas glands from pigs and cattle. Many people had allergic reactions to this insulin, however, so scientists began synthesizing insulin to make it more tolerable. To do this, they used a lot of genetic manipulation. First, they synthesized genes to create the two chains that compose an insulin molecule. Then they stitched them together into a bit of circular DNA known as a plasmid. Plasmids can be transferred between bacteria to pass along traits. (This is one of the ways bacteria transfer antibiotic resistance to each other.) In this case, the bacteria passed along the ability to make insulin. For many years, the insulin that people with diabetes were taking was made by genetically manipulated E. coli. Today, most people use recombinant human insulin, which is produced by E. coli or yeast.

You don't hear many people protesting the genetic modifications used to make insulin drugs. Why are we are so much more inclined to complain when these techniques are used to improve our food? What is it about food that makes us so irrational?

More disturbing than our irrationality about GMOs is that it seems to be having an effect on food policy. In 2016, Vermont became the first U.S. state to require food labels to show whether or not the food contains GMOs. Cheese was exempted from this law (Vermont is a big cheese producer), as was meat from animals that ate GMO feed. State lawmakers didn't want to hurt local businesses, after all—just the big, bad food companies.

Many companies understandably hated this law and began

to refuse to sell their products in Vermont. But others tried to comply—and in the process revealed even bigger flaws in the state's policy.

Rather than create different labels for the products they sold in Vermont, some major food companies simply added this new GMO language to all their labels, regardless of where the foods were sold. But what if other states started imposing different labeling regulations on food companies? That would be a recipe for disaster. It would be hard enough for large companies with significant infrastructure and resources to comply. But it would be pretty much impossible for smaller companies to make this work.

A federal solution proved to be somewhat more palatable, even to those companies that opposed GMO labeling altogether. In July 2016, President Obama signed the National Bioengineered Food Disclosure Standard, which set nationwide criteria for labeling GMO foods and made all state labeling laws moot. But the law doesn't specify how some ingredients should be handled. For instance, if the oil in a product is extracted from a GMO food, that oil doesn't necessarily contain modified DNA. If it doesn't, it might not have to be labeled GMO, even though it comes from a genetically modified organism. The law also allows companies considerable discretion in how they identify GMO ingredients in their foods. Companies can simply present the information on the label, or they can include a QR code that sends consumers to a website that contains this information. Surely, few people will bother to visit the website, and even fewer will do it in the store as they're shopping.

I'm not the only person who recognizes the futility of this law, although not everyone shares my concern about the disturbing antiscientific impulses it represents. Many anti-GMO activists are angry about it, too. They think it is toothless, and they are right. In one of my favorite responses, Senator Bernie Sanders, who was at that time running for president (and who as a senator from Vermont supported the labeling of GMO foods), tweeted out a picture of a can of Coca-Cola next to a package of Peanut M&Ms. His text asked, "Can you tell from these photos which product contains GMOs?"

Sanders's intent was to mock the fact that the tiny text on the M&Ms and the QR code on the soda can wouldn't make it easier for anyone to know that these foods contained GMOs. But he chose candy and sugar-laden soda to make his point. Does anyone really need a label to know that neither of these foods is particularly healthy? People shouldn't be concerned about GMOs in the foods as much as about the foods themselves. Even if Coca-Cola and M&Ms were totally GMO-free, no one could claim they are good for you.

THE BOTTOM LINE

As a person who cares about facts, I'm hopeful that, as more and more evidence accumulates, public opinion about GMO safety will change. Perhaps one of the most convincing pieces of evidence came out in 2016, when the National Academies of Sciences, Engineering, and Medicine published what seems to me to be the most comprehensive review of GMO safety ever performed. I'd encourage you to read it, but it's 388 pages long, and most of you have better ways to spend your time. So here's the gist.

Yes, there's a lot of controversy surrounding GMOs, but the evidence we have shows they are as safe to eat as conventional foods. It's possible that changes to the DNA of plants in the future could result in new allergies to foods, but we haven't seen that yet, and allergies exist with conventional foods, too.

What GMOs haven't done yet, though, is boost production

in such a way as to increase yields massively. In other words, they haven't yet achieved Borlaug's dream of feeding the world. They've helped farmers by making it easier to raise crops and fight off pests, but modifications that might make crops grow faster or better haven't yet fully succeeded.

GMOs arguably do have some environmental downsides to them. For instance, herbicide-resistant crops have enabled farmers to use more herbicides to control weeds in their fields. This has led to the development of "superweeds" that are resistant to herbicides—just like the crops the farmers are trying to protect. No one should be under the delusion that just because GMOs are safe to eat, we can't screw things up by tinkering with the genetic codes of the organisms with which we share this planet.

Now you don't have to read the report. You're welcome.

Despite the many arguments and studies showing that GMOs are safe, there are legitimate arguments about what GMOs mean for the balance of power in the food industry. According to the U.S. Supreme Court ruling in *Diamond v. Chakrabarty* (1980), genetically modified organisms can be patented. This means that GMO seeds usually sold by large food companies can be heavily restricted and controlled. In the old days, farmers would save a certain amount of their crops to produce seeds for the next year's planting. With practice, they could become self-sustaining and save money that would otherwise be needed to purchase seeds. Now, thanks to GMO patents and the laws that enforce them, food companies can make farmers sign agreements saying they will use the seeds only for a single season and won't save them for the next year. These companies can also test crops that farmers are growing and sue them if they're using the corporation's seeds without permission. This dystopian scenario is common currency among anti-GMO activists, and while it has actually happened far fewer times than the Internet might have you believe, it has happened.

These problems are the result of imperfect farming and the laws that regulate agribusiness, not of GMOs themselves. Genetically modified organisms are far more benign than most people recognize. There's no evidence suggesting that eating GMOs raises the risk of food allergies, negatively impacts our gastrointestinal tract, or messes with our DNA in any way. Eating them isn't related to the development of cancer, autism, obesity, kidney disease, or any other disease. Foods that contain GMOs aren't inherently unhealthy, any more than are foods that don't contain them. The companies that are trying to sell you foods by declaring them "GMO-free!" are using the absence of GMOs to their advantage — not yours.

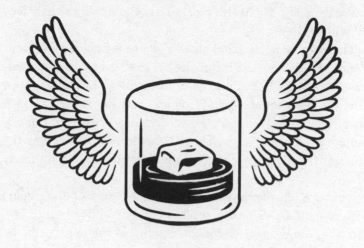

ALCOHOL

I LOVE scotch. I have a hard time explaining that to people who don't. My wife, who falls into the "don't" camp, thinks ten-year-old Laphroaig smells like cough syrup. I think it smells like heaven. But to each their own.

One evening not long ago, I was enjoying a bit of scotch in our sunroom, contentedly reflecting upon the fading light outside the window and the heavenly warmth inside my glass, when my oldest child walked in and told me I was going to die.

When I collected myself and asked him why, he said, "Because you're drinking. My health teacher at school told us that alcohol will kill you."

There's no question that alcohol abuse is unbelievably dangerous. But that doesn't mean alcohol itself is bad. In fact, medical studies have linked it to a number of health benefits. To be sure, the news about alcohol isn't *all* good, nor is the evidence in its favor enough to start recommending its use. But there is enough evidence to suggest that I should be able to enjoy the occasional scotch in my sunroom without fearing my untimely death.

This was not the first time I would find myself disagreeing with my children's health teachers, nor would it be the last. My wife, Aimee, a wise woman, convinced me to drop the issue rather than fight with the teacher — or our son — about it.* But for my sake, and for his, I have to set the record straight. Otherwise, he might grow up to fear alcohol rather than have a healthy respect for its risks — and an appreciation of its rewards, of which there are more than you might think.

WHAT WE KNOW ABOUT ALCOHOL AND HEALTH

Alcohol is controversial, and there are a lot of studies out there about it. I'll review the best of them quickly but in some detail, so you know I'm not cherry-picking the most upbeat evidence and burying the bad stuff.

Research into the effects of alcohol consumption on health has been going on for a long time, but the past few decades have seen the strongest studies. An epidemiologic study published

---

* The teachers aren't totally off the hook. I'm going to buy them all copies of this book.

in 1990, for instance, included results from more than 275,000 men whom researchers had followed since 1959. Compared to the subjects who never drank alcohol, the men in the study who consumed one to two drinks a day had a significantly reduced risk of death from both coronary heart disease and "all causes" — meaning death by any means. (Studies that look at risk sometimes examine death from a specific cause — in this case, heart disease — and death overall. It's the result regarding death overall that's more powerful. After all, if an intervention makes it less likely that you will die from a specific cause, just to let you die from some other cause at the same time, the intervention hasn't really done you much good.)

If you believe the results of this observational study, you'll conclude that people who drink moderately (for men, that means one to two drinks a day) are likely to live longer. People who consume three or more drinks a day (a rate that most experts consider "heavy" drinking) are at a lower risk of death from coronary heart disease but a higher risk of death overall.

A 2004 observational study came to similar conclusions. It followed about 6,600 men and 8,000 women for five years and found that, compared with people who didn't drink at all and those who had more than two drinks a day, people who consumed about one drink a day on average had a lower rate of death.

Results like these have been consistent across a number of studies. Even a study published in the gloomily titled journal *Alcoholism: Clinical and Experimental Research* agrees that moderate drinking seems to be associated with a decreased risk of death overall.

According to these and other studies, almost all of the major benefits of drinking seem to have to do with staving off cardiovascular disease. Men in particular seem to be able to consume a surprisingly large amount of alcohol — more than the vast majority of people can drink — while still obtaining this protective effect.

When it comes to cancer, the picture isn't as rosy. A 2007 study involving the Women's Health Study cohort found that increased alcohol consumption was associated with an increased risk of breast cancer. More broadly, a 2014 systematic review of research on the connection between alcohol and breast cancer found that the overall consensus is that each additional drink per day increases the relative (not absolute) risk of breast cancer by 2%. Although this is a statistically significant increase, it's still small — suggesting that alcohol contributes very little to women's overall absolute risk of breast cancer.

Similar evidence has been found for a connection between alcohol and other types of cancer. A meta-analysis of studies tracking alcohol intake and the incidence of colorectal cancer found that heavy drinkers (but not light or moderate drinkers) were at increased risk of that disease. Other studies found no relationship with respect to bladder cancer or ovarian cancer. One study that included all cancers found that light drinking was protective, moderate drinking had no effect, and heavy drinking was detrimental.

To recap: Moderate alcohol consumption seems not to significantly increase your risk for cancer, and it appears to safeguard your cardiovascular health. It's been associated with other benefits as well. A cohort of about 6,000 people followed in Britain found that those who consumed alcohol at least once a week had significantly better cognitive function in middle age than those who did not drink at all. This protective effect on cognition was seen in people who consumed up to thirty drinks a week — more than four drinks a day on average.*

---

* That's a lot of alcohol, and more than anyone I know would recommend.

Cognition and cardiovascular health aren't the only ways in which alcohol might help rather than hurt you. A 2004 systematic review found that moderate drinkers had lower rates of diabetes (up to 56% lower) compared with nondrinkers. Heavy drinkers, it should be noted, had an increased incidence of diabetes.

This is all good news for scotch lovers — but savvy readers should be asking for still more evidence. After all, what about randomized controlled trials? Epidemiologic evidence and associations take us only so far; they don't prove causation. Only randomized controlled trials can do that.

In 2015, such a trial was published in the *Annals of Internal Medicine,* the influential journal of the American College of Physicians. The organizers of the study randomized patients with well-controlled type 2 diabetes to drink 150 milliliters (a little over half a cup) of either water, white wine, or red wine with dinner for two years. (The beverages were provided to patients free of charge, which in my opinion is better compensation than participants in most studies receive.) The subjects were all placed on a Mediterranean diet, getting lots of vegetables, olive oil, and protein (especially fish), with no calorie restrictions.

When the researchers assessed their subjects after two years, they found that the trial subjects who had been assigned to drink wine appeared to be healthier than those who had been stuck with water. The subjects who got wine, most notably red wine, showed a reduction in cardiometabolic risk factors — those for heart disease, diabetes, or stroke. Furthermore, none of the subjects who'd had wine showed any significant adverse effects from drinking the alcohol.

In another analysis of the same study, the most interesting finding was about blood pressure. While the subjects' overall twenty-four-hour blood pressure didn't vary between groups, those in the red wine group had periods of the day during which their blood pressure improved versus those who drank water. In some cases, this effect was more pronounced in subjects with specific genotypes — that is, people whose particular genetic makeup caused them to metabolize alcohol faster. Again, the alcohol caused no significant adverse effects. I should note that this contradicts the findings of a systematic review of epidemiologic studies showing that alcohol intake may be associated with a small but significant increase in blood pressure. But as I've discussed many times, you should almost always trust randomized controlled trials above observational studies.

Typical of cutting-edge dietary health research, there are some studies that seem to contradict or at least temper these findings. For instance, a shorter-term trial looking at red wine consumption found that it had no effect, positive or negative, on blood pressure in patients with atherosclerosis, or a buildup of plaque in their arteries. It did result in improved cholesterol levels, however, even though many patients were already being treated with statins, drugs that work to lower the amount of cholesterol in the blood. And a 2011 meta-analysis that examined sixty-three controlled trials of wine, beer, and spirits found that all of these beverages increased levels of HDL cholesterol (the "good" cholesterol). There was even a dose response, meaning that the more alcohol the subjects consumed, the greater the effect seemed to be.

Taken together, all of this evidence points to a few conclusions. First, the majority of the research suggests that moderate alcohol consumption is associated with decreased rates of cardiovascular disease, diabetes, and death. Second, it also seems to be associated with increased rates of some cancers (especially breast cancer), cirrhosis, chronic pancreatitis, and accidents, although this negative impact from alcohol seems to be smaller than its positive impact on cardiovascular health. Indeed, the gains in cardiovascular disease seem to outweigh the losses in all the other diseases combined. The most recent report of the USDA Scientific Advisory Panel agrees that "moderate alcohol consumption can be incorporated into the calorie limits of most healthy eating patterns."

There's a lot more work to do on this front. For one thing, the studies I've mentioned cover a variety of different kinds of alcohol. We need more research targeted to specific types of alcohol before we can say with certainty that *all* alcohol can have positive effects when consumed in moderation. Although many studies have focused on wine, fewer have looked at beer or hard liquor in isolation. Many people with chronic illnesses also wonder whether alcohol is as safe for them, or as potentially beneficial, as for healthy individuals. Unfortunately, most studies haven't been that specific.

THE EVIDENCE AGAINST MODERATE DRINKING DOESN'T STAND UP TO SCRUTINY

If the research about alcohol makes one thing clear, it's that you can enjoy a drink once in a while without worrying about negatively impacting your health. To the contrary, you're probably helping it.

Of course, if you tell your friends at a cocktail party that you've read that alcohol isn't bad for you, let alone that it might actually be good for you, someone there is inevitably going to argue with you. If they're reasonably well-informed, they may even cite a study from 2016 that led to a spate of news stories proclaiming that "a little alcohol may not be good for you after all." Many news reports used these exact words to describe the study's results.

For all the attention it received, this study wasn't a new trial or experiment. It was an updated systematic review and meta-analysis that excluded a lot of research that its authors — who published their results in the *Journal of Studies on Alcohol and Drugs* — declared was flawed. The main problem, they argued, was that many of the previous studies lumped people who used to drink, but no longer did so, in with people who never drank. They further asserted that many of these people might actually have quit drinking because they were sick and were told to give up alcohol. This meant that these sick ex-drinkers were being counted as abstainers in the studies, biasing the results in a way that would make drinking moderately look healthier than not drinking at all. Because their study excluded these ostensibly biased results, the authors argued that they presented a more accurate depiction of the connection between alcohol and health than prior research on the subject had.

They also looked only at studies that examined all death from all causes considered together. Of the eighty-seven studies they found that met this criterion, only thirteen strictly made sure that lifetime abstainers (and not quitters) were the reference group. When the authors looked at those thirteen studies and compared lifetime abstainers with everyday drinkers, they didn't find any statistically significant difference between the groups. Those who drank at least 65 grams of alcohol a day (about 4.5 drinks) did, however, have an increased risk of death.

The researchers went on to exclude the "lesser-quality studies," and to consider only seven. The results were unchanged. They then excluded one more study that had results heavily favoring alcohol. The remaining six studies suggested that people who consumed two to three drinks a day had a slightly elevated risk of death. But those who consumed one to two drinks, as well as those who consumed three to four and a half drinks, did not have an elevated risk. When it comes to observational research, that's a pretty weak finding. But that conclusion somehow made the headlines.

If you look closely at the review, it's clear that the authors excluded a lot of studies that seem to have already taken into account their concerns. For instance, one study I discussed earlier in this chapter looked at all-cause mortality for subjects 55 to 65 years old. After researchers controlled for prior drinking as well as other confounding factors, they found that the subjects who drank a moderate amount of alcohol had a lower risk of death than either abstainers or heavy drinkers. They also cited five earlier studies that accounted for the "former drinker" problem, yet still found the protective effect of light to moderate drinking against all-cause mortality. It's unclear to me why these studies didn't factor into the updated systematic review and meta-analysis published in the *Journal of Studies on Alcohol and Drugs.*

That doesn't mean these authors did anything wrong. Researchers always have to make judgment calls about what to include in a meta-analysis. But the authors didn't clearly explain why they made the judgment calls they did.* That makes me concerned that they might have been cherry-picking.

It's also important to recognize another limitation of the systematic review and meta-analysis: it looked only at all-cause mortality and found no benefit of alcohol consumption. As we've seen in randomized controlled trials and other studies cited in this chapter, that finding doesn't preclude a benefit in terms of cardiovascular events such as heart attack or process measures such as blood pressure or cholesterol levels. A 2011 meta-analysis, for example, looked at mortality from a va-

---

* For the record, I've had email conversations with one of the authors, who believes that he did explain those calls well. We have to agree to disagree.

riety of cardiovascular causes. The researchers who conducted this meta-analysis also performed a sub-analysis that classified former drinkers appropriately. They found that both with and without this adjustment, active drinkers had a lower incidence of, and a lower mortality from, a variety of cardiovascular diseases. In the same vein, other studies have found associations between alcohol consumption and better cognitive function, lower rates of diabetes, and improved blood lipids. (The story for cancer is much more mixed.)

Individual randomized controlled trials not included in the updated systematic review and meta-analysis back up and extend its findings, suggesting that moderate drinking can help stave off diabetes and improve blood pressure and cholesterol levels. There's even that meta-analysis of sixty-three controlled trials, mentioned earlier in this chapter, showing alcohol's positive effects on HDL cholesterol. Anyone who claims that alcohol has no health benefits needs to reckon with findings like these.

At best, then, the 2016 systematic review and meta-analysis shows no evidence that anyone consuming two or fewer alcoholic drinks a day is at a higher *or* a lower risk of dying. At worst, the authors left out trials that showed a benefit. No matter how you slice it, this is good news for moderate drinkers.

ALCOHOL IS *DEFINITELY* A PROBLEM WHEN YOU ABUSE IT

None of this is to say that alcohol can't be a problem, or that we should ignore its abuse when talking about the health effects of alcohol. Drinking too much alcohol is bad for you, and you shouldn't do it. Period.

Alcohol abuse and alcoholism can be defined in many different ways, but the simplest is when a person's drinking starts to hurt his or her relationships, physically or psychologically harm him or her, or negatively affect his or her quality of life. Moderate drinking — often defined as up to one drink a day on average for women and up to two drinks a day for men — typically does not earn someone a diagnosis of alcoholism, but anything more than that will set off alarm bells for most health care professionals. The differences between men and women are mostly because of size (on average), relative levels of fat, and even perhaps genetics.

In the research world, there is often a fine — but very bright — line between healthy drinking and dangerous drinking. Consider the example of the United States.

Alcohol consumption — and the system of cultural norms that governs it — varies from country to country. Philip J. Cook used data from the National Epidemiologic Survey on Alcohol and Related Conditions to examine alcohol use in the United States. In his book *Paying the Tab*, Cook explains that Americans drink far less alcohol overall than many people assume, but those who drink too much, drink *way* too much.

If you live in the United States and have two alcoholic drinks every three months, you're likely in the top half of alcohol consumers in the country. Thirty percent of Americans drink no alcohol whatsoever. None. The next 10% consume, on average, about one drink a year. The next 10% consume about seven drinks a year. This amount of alcohol — less than one drink per month — is negligible, and half of Americans drink less than that.

Even if you're in the top 50% of drinkers, you might hardly be drinking at all. The next 10% drink, on average, less than a drink a week. The 10% after that (between the 60th and 70th percentiles) consume two drinks a week. To remain in the eighth decile (between the 70th and 80th percentiles), you still have to drink less than one drink a day.

But then it gets interesting.

Those in the ninth decile (between the 80th and 90th percentiles) consume, on average, fifteen drinks a week, or just a bit more than two drinks a day. Most of these people are what experts call "social drinkers," a category that the National Institute on Alcohol Abuse and Alcoholism defines differently for men and women. For women, it means consuming no more than seven drinks a week and three on any one day. For men, it's no more than fourteen drinks a week and four on any one day.

Keep in mind that the best studies about alcohol and health tend to agree that one to two drinks a day is fine for your health, maybe even beneficial. What this means for social drinkers is that even if they're drinking more than 80% of their compatriots, their alcohol consumption might not be a problem. It's a lot more alcohol than the rest of Americans are drinking, but it's still in the range of okay.

It's in that last decile that things go off the rails. Whereas people in the ninth decile consume fifteen drinks a week, people in the tenth and final decile have seventy-four drinks a week on average. *Seventy-four!* You have to average two bottles of wine a day just to make it into the bottom half of this decile. I don't need to refer you to the health studies from earlier in the chapter to give you a sense of how destructive this kind of drinking is. Seventy-four drinks a week is more than four and a half bottles of scotch. It's three cases of beer. It's ten beers every day — on average.

Consuming this much alcohol may seem extreme, and it is. But we're talking about 24 million people here. These 10% of Americans drink more than half of all the alcohol consumed in the United States every year. They're not healthy; far from it. They suffer from a range of health problems, from cirrhosis to diabetes to cancer. And they're spending a whole lot of money on alcohol itself. If those 10% could reduce their drinking to the level of the ninth decile, overall alcohol sales in the United States would fall by 60%.

If social drinking defines the ninth decile of American drinkers, binge drinking characterizes the tenth — and it's deadly. Moreover, to be a binge drinker, you don't have to be in the tenth decile; you can be in the ninth decile, or even below it. You just need to concentrate your alcohol intake into fewer days. Recall that people in the ninth decile consume an average of fifteen drinks a week, or just over two drinks a day. That's an average. You can drink all fifteen drinks on Saturday night, drink nothing for the rest of the week, and still qualify as both a member of the ninth decile and a binge drinker.

Binge drinking, defined as four or more drinks on a single occasion for women and five or more drinks for men, isn't rare either. More than 17% of all Americans are binge drinkers, and more than 28% of people ages 18 to 24 are. Binge drinking is most prevalent among Americans who have a household income of at least $75,000. In the United States, at least, this makes binge drinking a solidly middle-class problem, rather than an issue that affects poorer citizens (as many people assume).

Alcohol abuse is a huge problem — for both individuals and society. A 2012 Centers for Disease Control and Prevention report based on 2010 data found that binge drinking accounted for about half of the more than 80,000 deaths due to alcohol that occurred in the United States that year. The CDC estimated the economic costs associated with excessive alcohol consumption in the United States to be about $225 billion dollars. Alcohol misuse isn't connected only to health, income, and age; it's also linked to crime. The National Council on Alcoholism and Drug Dependence reports that alcohol use is a factor in 40% of all violent crimes in the United States, including 37% of rapes and 27% of aggravated assaults. Crime and alcohol are an especially toxic combination among young people. A recent study in the journal *Pediatrics* investigated the factors associated with death in youths who get into trouble with the law. The researchers found that about 19% of delinquent males and 11% of delinquent females misused alcohol. Further, they found that even five years after detention, those with an alcohol problem had a 4.7 times greater risk of death from external causes, such as homicide, than those without this problem.

Of course, even young people whom most of us wouldn't call "delinquent" can get into trouble — health-wise and otherwise — when they binge drink. In 1995 alone, more than 460,000 alcohol-related incidents of violence were reported on college campuses in the United States. A 2014 prospective study found that college students were more likely to commit both psychological and physical dating abuse on days they drank alcohol. A 2016 report on colleges and drinking noted that every year more than 1,800 college students die from alcohol-related accidents. About 600,000 are injured while under alcohol's influence, almost 700,000 are assaulted, and almost 100,000 are sexually assaulted. About 400,000 have unprotected sex, and 100,000 are too drunk to know whether they consented.

What's more, young users can easily find their alcohol intake spinning out of control. About 15% of the people who use alcohol in college eventually become dependent, meaning they have a higher tolerance to alcohol, and potentially also experience withdrawal when they don't consume it. From there, it's only a small step to addiction.

As of this writing, alcohol is arguably the most dangerous drug in the world. An oft-quoted (and hotly debated) study in the UK medical journal the *Lancet* reflected as much. It ranked drugs according to their "harm score," both to users and to others. Alcohol was clearly the worst.

You could make a case that heroin, crack cocaine, and methamphetamine would be more harmful than booze if they were legal and more commonly used, but the fact remains: alcohol is incredibly easy to come by and abuse, and doing so is extremely dangerous. If someone is too young to manage their drinking responsibly, or if they are addicted to alcohol, they should absolutely steer clear of it. The modest health benefits of drinking a moderate or small amount of alcohol pale in comparison with the harm that can come from drinking too much.

PREGNANCY AND ALCOHOL

In addition to young people and alcoholics, pregnant women are often urged to abstain from alcohol completely. This is mainly because of the risk of fetal alcohol spectrum disorders (FASDs), a group of physical and cognitive problems that result from women drinking while their fetuses are developing. The vast majority of women I know follow this advice and drink zero alcohol during pregnancy — not wine, not beer, nothing.

I won't argue here that pregnant women should drink during pregnancy or that they shouldn't. I'll just say this: Most of the research that links alcohol to problems in pregnancy is looking at binge drinking. There's relatively little evidence to support a link between light or even moderate drinking and FASDs. Women in Europe don't abstain completely from alcohol consumption while they are pregnant. Some studies show that more than twice as many (or more) pregnant women drink there than in the United States, without corresponding increases in FASDs.

It's not hard to find studies that link alcohol consumption to childhood development disorders, but for practically every one of these studies, you can find another in which the links are weak, if they're there at all. For instance, a large cohort study in Denmark — where social norms about drinking during pregnancy are more lax than in the United States—found "weak" and "inconsistent" evidence linking binge drinking during pregnancy to the executive functions of children who resulted from those pregnancies. The researchers found no links at all between low to moderate consumption and later physical or psychological problems.

On the other end of the spectrum is one of the most cited studies on this subject, which did find a link between most levels of alcohol consumption and problems in pregnancy. More than five hundred pairs of parents and children were studied to learn about alcohol use during pregnancy. About a quarter of the women denied any use, 64% reported low use, and 13% reported moderate or heavy use. Children born to mothers with any alcohol use were found to have more behavioral problems and delinquent behavior than those whose mothers didn't drink at all.

However, the study also found that the women who drank during pregnancy were also more likely to have (or have kids with) "higher lead levels, higher maternal age, and lower education level, prenatal exposure to cocaine and smoking, custody changes, lower socioeconomic status, and paternal drinking and drug use at the time of pregnancy." Any of these factors, in addition to or apart from the alcohol, might help explain the babies' abnormal development.

If you're confused by this contradictory evidence, you're not alone. Even the doctors who should know the most about the dangers of drinking while pregnant seem to be conflicted. A study published in 2010 surveyed obstetricians to see what their knowledge, opinions, and practices were regarding their patients' use of alcohol. I was shocked to learn that only 47% thought the relationship between alcohol and fetal development was clear; 46% thought it wasn't.

When I talk to doctors about this issue, I find that their public and private stances are often very different. Publicly (especially in conversations with patients), they are much more likely to say that no amount of alcohol is safe for pregnant women. Privately, they will almost always admit that there's pretty much no evidence showing that the occasional drink is going to harm a baby in utero.

Doctors don't trust the public with such nuance. Better to be safe than sorry, they think. But I'm going to hold you to a higher standard.

While there are no absolutes in life, there is very little solid evidence that light drinking during pregnancy will harm a developing fetus. This is especially true after the first trimester. Emily Oster, an economist at Brown University and a former pregnant woman, reviewed the evidence in her book, *Expecting Better,* and concluded that one to two drinks a week in the first trimester and up to a drink a day in the second and third trimesters is safe. Based on her research, she advises pregnant women not to consume shots (which can easily lead to overdrinking and spikes in blood alcohol levels) and not to drink a lot at any one time. That's sensible, too.

Ultimately, pregnant women need to make their own decisions about alcohol and pregnancy. I won't judge them for abstaining, nor will I judge them for having a glass of wine every now and then.

THE BOTTOM LINE

Some people should not drink. If you're taking a drug that reacts badly with alcohol, or if you can't keep your consumption to a healthy level, you need to avoid alcohol altogether. Even if you're not in one of these groups, I wouldn't go so far as to tell you to start drinking because alcohol is good for you. That's rarely the conclusion of any studies about alcohol, no matter how positive the results. Nor is it the advice of any doctors I know.

But if you're a healthy person who drinks alcohol responsibly, you can feel confident that you're not doing yourself any harm. In fact, you may actually see some benefits from your light or moderate alcohol consumption.

Since alcohol is a potent substance and very easy to misuse, I'm going to do something here that I do nowhere else in this book. I'm going to block quote from the most recent USDA guidelines, which—when it comes to this subject—are worth keeping in mind:

> If alcohol is consumed, it should be in moderation—up to one drink per day for women and up to two drinks per day for men—and only by adults of legal drinking age. For those who choose to drink, moderate alcohol consumption can be incorporated into the calorie limits of most healthy eating patterns. The *Dietary Guidelines* does not recommend that individuals who do not drink alcohol start drinking for any reason; however, it does recommend that all foods and beverages consumed be accounted for within healthy eating patterns.

See? Don't take it from me. If you enjoy the occasional scotch, don't let anyone—not even your own child or his or her health teacher—convince you that you're doing something wrong. In more ways than you think, you may be doing yourself a favor.

Eight

COFFEE

I DON'T like to eat breakfast before I leave for work. It's not that I dislike breakfast food; it's just that I'm not hungry early in the morning. But while I regularly forgo the meal itself, I simply can't do without my morning cup of coffee.

I love coffee. I love the taste. I love the ritual. For a couple of years, I was even into roasting my own coffee beans at home. Roasting coffee can be done in a machine that's sort of like an air-based popcorn popper. It's not as hard to roast coffee beans as you might think, but the smell can be pretty bad, and it releases a lot of smoke. After I set off our smoke alarm for the second time while our young kids were asleep, my wife banned me from using the machine in the house, and my enjoyment of home-roasted coffee came to an end.

Without question, there's never been a better time in history to drink coffee. So many varieties are available. The coffee you get from a pod machine like a Keurig—and which is so close to "instant" that it may as well be—is of a quality that would have been nigh on impossible to brew so easily at home years ago. Even where I live in Indiana, a state that is not known for its coffee scene, I can go a few blocks in any direction from my office and find a couple of places to buy an excellent cup.

Amazingly, given how delicious and ubiquitous coffee is, some people think it's unhealthy. For one thing, it contains caffeine, which is a psychoactive drug—a fact that might lead you to conclude it can be abused. Many people consider caffeine to be habit-forming and talk about people who consume it as if they were addicts. But fears about coffee go beyond that. Coffee has long had a reputation as being seriously unhealthy. Health-related bans on coffee can be found dating back to the sixteenth century, and modern authorities have continued this trend. In 1991, for example, the World Health Organization labeled coffee as possibly carcinogenic. Still other fears abound. Some people genuinely think that coffee can dehydrate you, for instance, or can negatively impact the development of growing children, or that too much of it can be bad for your heart.

Not only are these fears of coffee simply unfounded, but they also overlook all the good attributes of coffee—besides its delicious flavor, I mean. In almost every respect, coffee's bad reputation gets the drink completely wrong. In fact, it has a surprising number of potential health benefits and few risks, if indeed any at all.

COFFEE WILL NOT STUNT YOUR KID'S GROWTH

Have you ever had a hot, steaming cup of Postum? This caffeine-free, roasted-grain beverage was once pushed by cereal magnate C. W. Post as a "healthy" alternative to coffee. In 1912, he produced an "instant" version that he heavily marketed with a bizarre and menacing slogan — "There's a reason" — which ran in ads that described people whose mental and/or physical health declined after drinking coffee. In one of my favorite ads, which ran on a full page of the March 1933 issue of the *American Magazine,* a teacher stands over a boy alone in a classroom. It begins, "Held back by coffee... this boy never had a fair chance." It goes on to say:

> "A dunce" they call him ... "a sluggard" they say. But Science lifts a hand in his behalf and says "You're wrong!"
>
> Put the blame on the real culprit ... pin the blame on coffee. Yes — *coffee!* For thousands of parents are giving their children coffee, and coffee harms children mentally — and physically.

The text continues for eleven more paragraphs about the evils of coffee and caffeine. It cites huge studies from "a world famous research institute" finding that less than 16% of kids who drank coffee got good marks versus 45% of those who did not. Another study showed that 85% of malnourished kids were drinking coffee daily. I'd love to see this research, but I've never been able to find it — probably because, in all likelihood, it doesn't exist.

Coffee has been demonized in cultures around the world for hundreds of years based on the belief that it's bad for our health. Post's marketing campaign is just one example of this fearmongering, though undoubtedly the most lucrative. It also had an outsize effect on coffee's reputation in the United States.

When I was a kid in the 1970s, my parents didn't think coffee would hurt me mentally, as Post had claimed, but they did worry that it would stunt my growth. They had a couple of reasons for this concern. Animal and laboratory studies had shown that high levels of caffeine were associated with increased calcium excretion (higher levels of calcium in the urine), and people figured this was depriving growing kids of the calcium they needed for bone development. Moreover, kids who drank coffee were thought to drink less milk, which had to mean they wouldn't grow as well — right?

As I got older, new research began showing that these concerns were overblown. For instance, a 1993 study that reviewed the existing evidence found that while it was true that short-term calcium excretion increased when people consumed caffeine, the body quickly compensated for the loss of calcium (that same day!) by decreasing calcium excretion, so that overall calcium levels remained unaffected. Another study, this one in 2002, expanded on those findings by considering how the theorized "decreased intake of milk" might come into play. Researchers determined that whatever negative effect drinking more coffee and less of other, calcium-containing beverages might cause would be offset by as little as one to two tablespoons of milk. They further noted that almost all the research confirming that coffee was linked to lower calcium was performed on people who were consuming less than an optimal amount of calcium.

Given that most of the people who are told that coffee will stunt their growth are healthy adolescents, these findings make such warnings seem pretty hollow. And there's more where those came from. A 1998 study followed eighty-one teenage girls over six years. The girls were divided into three groups by their intake of caffeine. There were no significant differences between the groups in their bone gain or bone health. Another study from two years earlier investigated whether there were differences in spine bone mineral content and density in participants' third decade of life based on their earlier diet. The researchers found that subjects who had consumed less calcium and protein had slightly lower bone density and mineral content, but that caffeine consumption made no difference at all.

In other words, there is absolutely no evidence that coffee will stunt your growth. But when I confronted my parents with this information as an adult, it barely slowed them down. They had another argument ready: "Coffee will dehydrate you!"

COFFEE WILL NOT DEHYDRATE YOU

There is a widespread belief that caffeine is a powerful diuretic, that it saps your body of fluid by making you pee more. Since you can become dehydrated when your fluid output outpaces your fluid intake, it stands to reason that coffee can make you dehydrated.

There is some research that supports this reasoning. In 2014, researchers from the United States and China published a meta-analysis of studies looking at healthy adults, coffee intake, and urine output. Combining the results of sixteen trials, these researchers found that people who drank 300 mg of caffeine experienced an increase in urine output of about 109 milliliters. Some studies looked only at a few hours after drinking the beverage, but about half followed people for twelve hours.

Now, you could use this research to argue that because coffee makes you urinate more, drinking it will eventually make you dehydrated unless you increase your intake of other fluids. But with a little context about the human body, this argument simply doesn't hold up.

First off, 100 milliliters or so really isn't that much urine. A healthy person can produce up to 2 liters of urine a day — twenty times that amount — if they're drinking enough. Plus, 300 mg of caffeine is the equivalent of three cups of coffee, at least as "cups" are defined by most studies.* If you're not drinking that much coffee, the dehydrating effect will be even lower.

Second, your body is exquisitely designed to prevent you from getting dehydrated. While caffeine might, in the short term, increase your urine output, your body will recognize the change and make adjustments to compensate. Much like your kidneys automatically decrease the amount of calcium you excrete after you consume coffee, they adapt to a higher output of urine by producing less urine in the hours after you consume caffeine, so that your overall fluid balance remains stable. As the authors of the 2014 study put it in their conclusion, "Concerns regarding unwanted fluid loss associated with caffeine consumption are unwarranted."

For the record, studies show that tea, which also contains caffeine, doesn't dehydrate people either. In fact, black tea was found to offer "similar hydrating properties to water." Carbonated beverages with caffeine also don't dehydrate you.

So caffeine won't dehydrate you, and it won't stunt your growth. What about the other big concerns people have about drinking coffee — that too much of it can give you cancer or be bad for your heart? As it turns out, the evidence shows exactly

---

* Pretty much all studies define a cup of coffee as an 8-ounce serving. That's smaller than what I imagine most people drink. A grande at Starbucks is 16 ounces, and I know many people who down at least two of those a day.

the opposite: on both counts, coffee seems to be shockingly good for you.

COFFEE IS LINKED TO A SURPRISING NUMBER OF HEALTH BENEFITS

In 2015, I agreed to write a column for the *New York Times* on the existing research about coffee and health. I assumed that I'd find some studies that associated coffee with good health outcomes and some that associated it with bad ones. That didn't turn out to be the case. Almost every study I found suggested there is a benefit to drinking coffee.

Research into the health benefits of coffee has been extensive, and the studies themselves are rather rigorous. Perhaps the most studies have focused on the connection between coffee consumption and cardiovascular health.

It makes sense that people would worry about what coffee does to your heart. After all, many a coffee drinker has had the unpleasant experience of drinking too much of the stuff and suffering a caffeine "overdose," which causes heart rates to rise and anxiety levels to spike.

As it turns out, however, drinking even fairly large amounts of coffee is probably *good* for your heart — and better than drinking none of it. There is research to prove this, and it's extensive. For instance, a 2014 systematic review and meta-analysis of research looking at long-term consumption of coffee and the risk of cardiovascular disease found thirty-six studies on this subject involving more than 1.27 million participants. That's a *huge* amount of research. The combined data show that subjects who consumed a moderate amount of coffee, about three to five cups a day, had the lowest risk of cardiovascular problems. Subjects who consumed five or more cups a day had no higher risk than those who consumed none.

This blew my mind. I couldn't understand how these results hadn't made front-page news.

And there was more. Just a few years before, in 2011, researchers published a meta-analysis looking at how coffee consumption might be associated with stroke, which is caused by problems with blood flow to the brain. The researchers found eleven studies that collectively included almost 480,000 participants. In these studies, the consumption of moderate amounts of coffee — in this case, two to six cups of coffee a day — was found to be associated with a lower risk of stroke than consuming no coffee at all. A meta-analysis published a year later, in 2012, confirmed these findings.

Another meta-analysis published the same year examined how drinking coffee might be associated with heart failure. Again, moderate consumption was associated with a lower risk of heart failure, with the lowest risk of all among those who consumed four cups of coffee a day. Subjects' coffee consumption had to get up to about *ten cups a day* before any bad associations could be seen.

These studies make clear that drinking moderate amounts of coffee is linked to lower rates of pretty much all cardiovascular disease. Even consumers on the very high end of the spectrum appear to have minimal, if any, ill effects.

But let's not cherry-pick. When it comes to coffee, after all, people worry about more than just heart health. For example, some people believe that coffee can cause cancer.

Certainly, some individual studies have found an association between coffee consumption and an increased risk of cancer, and as you might imagine, these findings cause a flurry of panic whenever the media picks them up. But when you look at them in the aggregate, most of these negative findings seem much less dire than they appear at first glance. For example, a meta-analysis published in 2007 found that increasing coffee consumption by two cups a day was associated with more than a 40% lower relative risk of liver cancer.* Two more-recent studies have confirmed these findings. Results from two meta-analyses looking at prostate cancer found that in the higher-quality studies examined, coffee consumption was not associated with negative outcomes related to this cancer either. The same holds true for breast cancer, where associations with coffee consumption were not statistically significant in two meta-analyses. A 2010 meta-analysis of studies on lung cancer did find an increasing risk as people's coffee consumption rose — but only among people who smoked. Drinking coffee may be protective for those who don't. What's more, the authors of that analysis warn that their results should be interpreted with caution because of the confounding (and likely overwhelming) health effects of smoking. A study looking at all cancers combined suggested that coffee might be associated with a reduced overall cancer incidence and that the more coffee you drink, the more protection it provides.

Beyond cancer and cardiovascular health, coffee seems to have a host of other protective properties. For one thing, it appears to promote liver health. A systematic review showed that drinking coffee was associated with improved liver function in subjects at risk for liver disease. In patients who already had liver disease, it was associated with a decreased progression to cirrhosis. In patients who already had cirrhosis, it was associated with a lower risk of death and a lower risk of developing liver cancer. The researchers also found that coffee consumption was associated with improved responses to antiviral therapy in patients with hepatitis C, as well as with better outcomes

---

* Yes, this is relative risk — not absolute risk — but 40% is nothing to sneeze at.

in patients with non-alcoholic fatty liver disease. They argue that daily coffee consumption should be encouraged — *encouraged!* — in patients with chronic liver disease.

And if all of that isn't enough, coffee may also help your brain. The most recent meta-analyses on neurologic disorders have found that coffee intake is associated with a lower risk of Parkinson's disease, lower cognitive decline in old age, and a potential protective effect against Alzheimer's disease.

Coffee might help protect against diabetes, too. A systematic review published in 2005 found that regular coffee consumption was associated with a significantly reduced risk of developing type 2 diabetes, with the lowest relative risk (about a third reduction in risk) for those who drank at least six or seven cups a day. A more recent study, published in 2014, included twenty-eight studies and more than 1.1 million participants. Again, the more coffee study subjects drank, the less likely they were to have diabetes.

In addition to these studies about the relationship between coffee consumption and specific diseases, some studies have looked at coffee and the risk of death from all causes. The news is good here, too. A meta-analysis published in 2014 reviewed twenty studies including almost a million people, and another, published in 2015, included seventeen studies containing more than a million people. Both found that drinking coffee was associated with a significantly reduced chance of death, period.

This is all great news for people who drink caffeinated coffee — but what about coffee that doesn't contain caffeine? As it turns out, there is one significant hole in the body of research about coffee, and this has to do with decaf. The study on diabetes and coffee intake mentioned previously included both caffeinated and decaffeinated coffee, but interestingly, most studies don't include data on the health impacts of decaf, perhaps because not enough people drink it. Overall, the data on decaf just aren't as comprehensive. There's less evidence overall for a potential benefit, but there's no evidence of any harmful associations either.

These inconclusive findings about decaffeinated coffee may make you wonder if it's the caffeine in coffee that provides a health benefit, rather than the coffee itself. To be honest, we don't know. It's possible that the exact cause varies from benefit to benefit. For instance, caffeine might help to slow or prevent neurologic problems by acting as a stimulant in the brain. This hypothesis is supported by the fact that decaffeinated coffee doesn't seem to be as protective as regular coffee in this regard, whereas tea is. When it comes to other diseases such as heart disease or liver disease, however, other caffeine-containing beverages don't seem to provide nearly the same benefit as coffee. (No one is arguing, for instance, that drinking diet soda might lower your chances of getting cancer.) What's more, decaffeinated coffee seems to have some of the same protective effects as regular coffee in areas other than the brain. Therefore, it's likely that something in coffee is good for us apart from its caffeine content. We just don't know what that something is.

While coffee appears to be beneficial when it comes to cancer, cognition, cardiovascular health, and diabetes, there are two metrics on which its effects seem to be less positive: blood pressure and cholesterol levels. Even in these two regards, however, it's likely that the claims about coffee's negative impacts are way overblown.

Given caffeine's effects on heart rate, some people have argued that it can't be good for those with high blood pressure, or even that it could *cause* high blood pressure in healthy people. A 2005 meta-analysis seemed to reinforce this argument when it found that in randomized controlled trials, ingestion of caffeine was associated with an increase in blood pressure. When the caffeine was from coffee, however, the blood pressure effect was small. A 2011 study found that caffeine intake could raise blood pressure for at least three hours. Again, there wasn't a significant relationship between long-term coffee consumption and higher blood pressure. Finally, a 2012 meta-analysis of ten randomized controlled trials and five cohort studies found no significant effect of coffee consumption on blood pressure or hypertension.

In addition to these blood pressure studies, two studies have shown that drinking unfiltered coffee can lead to increases in serum cholesterol levels and triglycerides—which (as I discussed in chapter 3) are markers for potential heart disease in people. Coffee that goes through a paper filter, however, seems to have the cholesterol-raising agent, known as cafestol, removed.

But how much do these ominous-sounding findings really matter? Blood pressure and cholesterol levels are process measures—that is, markers for diagnosable conditions. High blood pressure and high cholesterol are concerning to us because they can lead to disease or death. Disease and death are ultimately the things that matter most, and drinking coffee is associated with better outcomes in those domains.

I grant you that pretty much none of the research I've cited up to this point in this chapter consists of randomized controlled trials. It's important to remember that those types of studies are usually conducted to test whether what we are seeing in epidemiologic studies holds true. But most of us aren't drinking coffee because we think it will protect us. Most of us are worrying that it might be *hurting* us, and there's almost no evidence of that.

If any herb or vitamin had the kind of positive associations that coffee has across the board, the media would be all over it. They'd be pushing it on everyone. Whole interventions would be built around it. Instead, most of the media attention

I'd seen before I wrote my column for the *New York Times* in 2015 seemed to be negative. However, that sentiment appears to be changing. The newest USDA Dietary Guidelines, released in 2015, say that coffee is not only okay, but it also might be good for you. This was the first time the Dietary Guidelines Advisory Committee reviewed the effects of coffee on health. Ever.*

Of course, there's always the danger of going too far in the other direction. I'm not suggesting that we start serving coffee to little kids. Caffeine still has a number of effects parents might want to avoid in their children, including making them jittery and keeping them awake. Unborn children who are exposed to caffeine also might experience these effects — although this does not mean that pregnant women need to avoid coffee altogether. Far from it.

PREGNANT WOMEN CAN STILL DRINK COFFEE, JUST MAYBE NOT AS MUCH

In addition to the cautions about not giving coffee to kids, there are guidelines suggesting that pregnant women should not drink more than two cups a day. I know plenty of women who believe that, as with alcohol, any amount of caffeine is dangerous during pregnancy, and there is some evidence to support this belief. For instance, one 1997 study found an association between caffeine consumption and risk of miscarriage. The results of this and many other studies may be skewed, however. It turns out that women who drink a lot of caffeine are also more likely to smoke cigarettes and drink more than the nor-

---

* It appears that the USDA is agreeing with me more and more as time goes on. Maybe the staff there has been reading my columns.

mal amount of alcohol. These things could easily be confounding the relationship between caffeine and pregnancy.

Some women even worry about consuming caffeine *before* pregnancy—but they're probably worrying needlessly, too. Some of the headlines reporting evidence of this connection may be frightening, but a closer look at the studies themselves should reassure you. For example, one 2016 study published in the journal *Fertility and Sterility* followed 344 couples through the first seven weeks of gestation and found that women who consumed more than two caffeinated beverages *before* conception had a significantly higher chance of losing the pregnancy. But women who were pregnant by men who drank more than two caffeinated beverages a day also had an increased risk of miscarriage, by just about as much. Unless people are going to start arguing that coffee is bad for sperm (how is that even possible?), the lack of biological plausibility makes it more likely this is an association, not causation.

When we look at the evidence all together, as researchers did in a 2010 systematic review, we see that it doesn't make a strong case for a relationship between drinking coffee during pregnancy and bad outcomes for the baby. In fact, one randomized controlled trial even found that decreasing caffeine intake among pregnant women who were regular coffee drinkers did not significantly lower the risk of low birth weight or preterm birth.

Almost all the studies on pregnancy and coffee support the idea that drinking up to two cups of coffee a day is likely fine for pregnant women.* Although some studies support drink-

---

* Which is what the recommendations of the American College of Obstetricians and Gynecologists say (see http://www.acog.org/Resources-And-Publications/Committee-Opinions/Committee-on-Obstetric-Practice/Moderate-Caffeine-Consumption-During-Pregnancy). This is one of those instances where the official word seems to be based on research. We should acknowledge that!

ing three or even four cups a day, the evidence for that isn't as strong as it is for one to two cups.

So if your coffee consumption is within that range, stop worrying. You'll almost certainly be fine, as will your baby.

THE BOTTOM LINE

There's no evidence that coffee is bad for the average person. The data do not support the idea that we, collectively, are drinking too much of it, nor that coffee is associated with poor health outcomes. In fact, the opposite appears to be true. So don't let anyone tell you to avoid the stuff or insist that you need to cut down. Odds are you don't.

Fears about coffee seem to be subsiding slowly. My *New York Times* column, published in May 2015, was one of my most popular columns, and I received a huge amount of feedback on it, most of it (but certainly not all) positive.

One month later, the WHO reclassified coffee. After "reviewing more than 1000 studies in humans and animals," the organization found that "coffee drinking had no carcinogenic effects for cancers of the pancreas, female breast, and prostate, and reduced risks were seen for cancers of the liver and uterine endometrium." It now says that there is "inadequate evidence" to label coffee a carcinogen. When it comes to the WHO and cancer, that's about as good as it gets. An about-face on something like this is virtually unprecedented. The reclassification was correlated with my column, almost certainly not caused by it—but hey, a guy can dream, can't he?

To be clear, I am not arguing that you should start drinking coffee if you don't already, especially if you don't like it. Nor am I suggesting that if you already drink a moderate amount of coffee, you should start drinking it by the gallon. Too much of anything can be bad for you. And, of course, if you adulterate your coffee with all sorts of other ingredients such as creamers and sweeteners, the findings of the carefully crafted studies I've cited in this chapter go right out the window. While coffee itself may be healthy, that's not necessarily true of the added sugar and milk products.

It's time people stopped viewing coffee as something to be limited or avoided. It's a completely reasonable part of a healthy diet, and it appears to have more potential benefits than almost any other beverage we consume.

Coffee is more than my favorite breakfast drink; it's usually my breakfast, period. And I feel better about that now than ever before. It's time we started treating coffee as the wonderful elixir it is, not the witch's brew that C. W. Post made it out to be.

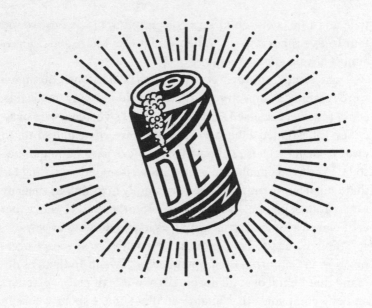

Nine

DIET SODA

I N addition to writing about food and nutrition in the course
of my career, I've delved into the research behind health
care reform, birth control, marijuana, and even circumci-
sion. I'm not afraid of a little controversy.

But no topic I've covered has been as polarizing as artificial
sweeteners. And no article I've written has been met with as
much anger and vitriol as the first piece I wrote on this subject
for the *New York Times,* in July 2015, in which I admitted, "My

wife and I limit our children's consumption of soda to around four to five times a week. When we let them have soda, it's . . . almost always sugar-free."

I was totally unprepared for the backlash. The comments were scathing. People argued that I should have my medical license revoked because I said that artificial sweeteners are okay. Others questioned whether I should have *my children taken away from me* because I allowed them the occasional sugar-free soda. I received emails and even handwritten letters telling me that I must be corrupt. People were simply incredulous that any sane, rational person — especially a doctor! — could believe that artificial sweeteners aren't killing us in any number of ways.

Things came to a head months later when an advocacy organization in California used open-access laws in Indiana to demand that I hand over all my emails about artificial sweeteners and any companies that might sell diet soda. I spent weeks in close contact with the lawyers for my university as they pulled, sifted through, and then packaged up my emails for release. I won't lie to you: it was a terrible violation of my privacy, and it ruined a month of my life — not because I was worried that the group would uncover some shady dealings with, or payoffs from, Big Soda, but simply because I don't like the idea of people reading my email.* Plus, my hilarious friends had started sending me emails asking whether "the big check from Pepsi" had arrived yet, and I knew the California watchdogs were going to have a field day.

In a way, these activists' concern is understandable; some "experts" on health and nutrition can be biased. Some months later, the *New York Times* broke a story about how the same type of subpoena the advocacy organization had used against me had revealed that a number of other scientists across the

---

* I'm not running for office, after all. And I never plan to.

country *did* have relationships, monetary and otherwise, with big food companies. But I wasn't part of that story, and I make no attempt to hide my biases — my love of scotch and black coffee, for instance, or my relationships with other researchers — in this book or in any of my other journalistic or academic writing.

Still, let me be explicit: I don't have any financial relationships with food companies. I don't consult for them. I don't exchange emails with them. I don't think I even know anyone who works for a big food company. I do have a famous friend who sometimes gets food or drink sent to him, and I think I've taken a few packs of gum for my kids from the pile in his office. I can't even remember what brand of gum it was — but knowing me, it was probably sugar-free, which means it contained an artificial sweetener.

I like to think that I've been as fair as possible in trying to determine which is worse for you: artificial sweeteners or sugar. But I make no apologies for my conclusions, which are based — as are all the other conclusions in this book — on research rather than anecdote, myth, emotion, or payola.

So let's talk about the research — and the problems with it. But before we get to that, it's important to understand what exactly sugar is, and what the class of nutrients it belongs to — carbohydrates — can do to our bodies.

CARBS AND OUR HEALTH

Carbohydrates, especially sugar, have become a real focus of concern for many nutrition professionals and laypeople alike. While some of that hatred is warranted, it doesn't mean you have to live your life carb-free in order to be healthy.

The major concern regarding carbohydrates is how they interact with and stimulate our insulin pathways. When we digest carbohydrates — molecules found in a plethora of foods, from fruits and grains to milk and starchy vegetables — the end result is glucose, which is released into the bloodstream. In a healthy person, insulin from the pancreas helps the body take glucose out of the blood and bring it into the cells, to be used as fuel for energy. Insulin also tells the fat cells to take glucose out of the bloodstream and store it as, well, fat. It acts as a feedback mechanism for the whole glucose regulation system. When there's more insulin around, the body is supposed to slow or stop the release of glucose into the bloodstream.

The problem arises when this process is pushed into overdrive. Many people believe that if you're consuming a lot of carbs, you're always putting glucose into your bloodstream, which keeps your body awash in insulin too much of the time. This leaves you primed for fat creation and storage, and can result in weight gain. It's not hard to find people these days who see a link between our past increase in carbohydrate consumption (as we shunned fat and the meat it often comes with) and the current obesity epidemic.

Increased carbohydrate consumption also might be related to the growing prevalence of type 2 diabetes. Type 1 diabetes develops when the pancreas can no longer produce insulin. When this happens, the body can't digest carbs appropriately, and blood glucose levels spike (hyperglycemia), which can be very dangerous. People with type 1 diabetes need to get insulin from outside sources, which allows them to use and store their glucose appropriately. But if they get too much insulin, they don't have enough glucose in the bloodstream to feed the brain and other organs (hypoglycemia). Therefore, people with type 1 diabetes need to monitor their glucose levels closely and give themselves just enough insulin to keep those levels in the proper range.

Type 2 diabetes is a different concern. In people with that condition, the pancreas may still be making insulin appropriately, but the body has become resistant to it. As I mentioned before, one of the things insulin does is to prevent the release of glucose into the bloodstream. When the liver becomes resistant to insulin, it doesn't listen well. It keeps releasing glucose, resulting in too much glucose in the bloodstream (again, hyperglycemia). Other things can go wrong as well, but it's important to understand this major difference: type 1 diabetes is when the body can't make insulin anymore; type 2 diabetes is when the body isn't responding to insulin appropriately.

Unlike type 1 diabetes, some type 2 diabetes is reversible. If physicians can get glucose levels, and the corresponding insulin levels, under control — often through dietary changes and weight loss — some people can regain their insulin sensitivity. Others cannot, and must be treated with medications that increase insulin to overcome the resistance, or increase sensitivity at the source.

People who have diabetes, or people who are at risk for it, watch their carbohydrate intake closely. This constant attention leads some people to think that carbohydrates *cause* diabetes, which just isn't the case. That said, carbohydrates can be a problem, especially when you're getting them in the form of sugar.

I'M NOT GOING TO DEFEND SUGAR

It's hard to defend sugar these days. For too long, companies have been adding it to foods in order to get people to eat them. They've also been caught — red-handed — trying to influence science by convincing researchers and doctors to malign fat and other nutrients while ignoring the dangerous effects of sugar.

In the mid-2010s, a postdoctoral researcher at the University of California, San Francisco, School of Dentistry named Cristin Kearns was digging through some archives when she stumbled upon a treasure trove of documents. They were from the 1960s, many of them originating with the Sugar Research Foundation. They included internal documents, historical reports, and statements concerning early debates about the dietary causes of congestive heart disease.

In 1965, the Sugar Research Foundation sponsored its first research project, published two years later in the *New England Journal of Medicine*. It argued that fats and cholesterol were the primary causes of congestive heart disease and that sucrose, or sugar, didn't really carry much risk. Given the focus of dietary advice over the decades that followed, this doesn't seem like it should have been that much of a surprise. It was, however, a much more contentious statement than you might think.

By the 1960s, there were two key theories regarding how nutrition affects heart disease. The first, fathered by Ancel Keys (remember the Minnesota Coronary Experiment from chapter 1?), argued that total fat, saturated fat, and cholesterol were to blame. The second, fathered by John Yudkin, argued that sugar was at fault. This was a war, and Keys's school of thought won out. But it may not have been a fair fight.

Along with the other documents Kearns unearthed in that neglected archive, she found correspondence between the Sugar Research Foundation and Roger Adams, a professor emeritus of organic chemistry at the University of Illinois, who served on the foundation's advisory board from 1959 to 1971. She also found correspondence between the foundation and Mark Hegsted, a professor of nutrition at the Harvard School of Public Health.

It seems that Yudkin's research was making the Sugar Research Foundation panic, so they proposed starting a new program to counter "negative attitudes towards sugar." In 1965, the foundation asked Fredrick Stare, the chair of the Department of Nutrition at the Harvard School of Public Health, to join its scientific advisory board.

On July 23, 1965, two days after a big *New York Herald Tribune* article highlighting the link between sucrose and heart disease, the Sugar Research Foundation approved Project 226.* Project 226 was a literature review by Hegsted and Robert McGandy, a colleague of Hegsted's, that was overseen by Stare. They were initially offered $500 and $1,000 ($3,800 and $7,500 today), respectively, for the project, but they eventually received a total of $6,500 ($48,900 today).

The Sugar Research Foundation provided them with articles that attacked sugar, likely so that they could contradict them. At every stage, the foundation stressed that it wanted the attacks on carbs debunked. The professors made it clear that they understood.

The work got delayed, because each time a new article attacking sugar came out, they had to revise their review to rebut the claims. The Sugar Research Foundation assessed the scientists' progress periodically. On November 2, 1966, the foundation told Hegsted, "Let me assure you this is quite what we had in mind and we look forward to its appearance in print."

Project 226 led to a two-part report published in the *New England Journal of Medicine* in 1967. It made no mention of the Sugar Research Foundation's funding of, or involvement in, the work. It consistently discounted results from nutritional studies, even those from randomized controlled trials that said fat reduction didn't work but sugar reduction did, and overstated the results of studies that said the opposite. And it concluded that there was "no doubt" that the only nutritional interven-

---

* I know this sounds like a conspiracy theory, but bear with me.

tions needed to prevent congestive heart disease were to reduce dietary cholesterol and substitute polyunsaturated fats for saturated fats.

It's rare that you get a smoking gun like the correspondence Kearns unearthed. It's clear that the funders of this research knew the results they wanted and the researchers understood this. Maybe the authors thought the results of their research were correct. But no one knew about their ties to the Sugar Research Foundation, and no one got to discuss the potential conflicts of interest until Kearns published her findings in 2016, about fifty years later — well after the damage was done.

We now know that the Harvard researchers got it wrong: consumed cholesterol does not pose nearly the danger that sugar does, and it's hard to argue that fats do either. Over the past few years, study after study has linked increased sugar intake to health problems. One study published in 2014, for instance, followed 11,733 people for almost fifteen years (163,039 person-years), during which 831 people died from cardiovascular disease. After controlling for other related factors, including sociodemographic ones, the researchers found that the top 20% of sugar consumers were more than twice as likely to die from heart disease as the bottom 20%. The accompanying editorial argued that drinking one 20-ounce Mountain Dew per day was enough to significantly increase a person's chances of dying from a cardiovascular event.

As with so many other things, the problem with sugar is that we've gone from thinking of it as something we might have once in a while to thinking it should be in all kinds of foods — or at least allowing food companies to put it there, a concession we make every time we buy a processed food that contains an excessive amount of sugar.*

---

* If this reminds you of what's happened with salt, it should. The problems are similar.

This has led critics to call for the banning of sugar or eliminating it completely from some people's diets. It's also caused people to begin to think that getting rid of sugar is the silver bullet we've all been waiting for. They even have research to prove it. For instance, a study published in 2016 claimed that lowering added sugar from about 30% of kids' daily calories to about 10% and replacing it with starch had led to impressive improvements in blood pressure, cholesterol levels, and insulin levels.

This study got a lot of press. It also led to some irrational exuberance in the media. But like so much nutrition research, it was lacking in many ways. First, the study took place over only nine days. Second, all of the food the kids ate was given to them free of charge, which likely resulted in other changes in their diets besides those in sugar intake. Finally, there was no control group.

I don't doubt that many kids, especially overweight or obese ones, would see improvements in their weight and health if they cut out many sources of sugar in their diets. But other changes could make a difference as well. And some sources of sugar are more problematic than others. Specifically, sugar that is added to foods is much worse for us than sugar that's found in foods naturally: a can of sweetened soda is worse than an apple.

We all know this intuitively, but it's worth considering why this is the case.

ADDED SUGAR IS THE *REAL* PUBLIC ENEMY NUMBER ONE

When medical professionals like me say "Sugar is bad for you," what we are really talking about is *added* sugar, not the naturally occurring sugars or carbohydrates you find in things like fruit.

The Centers for Disease Control and Prevention reports that American children are consuming between 282 (for girls) and 362 (for boys) calories of added sugar per day on average. This means that more than 15% of their caloric intake is from added sugar. Adults are doing slightly better, but not much (239 for women and 335 for men). This consumption isn't distributed equally across the population, though. For instance, about half of Americans consume no sugar drinks at all. The next 25% consume about 200 calories per day from sugar drinks. And the top 5% consume more than 560 calories a day from sugar drinks, or more than four 12-ounce cans of soda.

Consuming added sugar is significantly associated with being overweight or obese. A systematic review and meta-analysis published in 2013 examined thirty randomized controlled trials lasting at least two weeks and thirty-eight cohort studies lasting at least one year, all of which looked at how the intake of sugar was related to both adults' and children's weight. According to this review, the studies of adults that didn't restrict diet found that lowering the intake of added sugar led to people losing weight, and increasing the intake led to them gaining weight. The studies of children showed that those who had the highest intake of sugar-sweetened beverages (such as soda) were also significantly more overweight than those who had the lowest intake. Even though there were obviously many differences between these studies, the effects and relationships were consistent, even after eliminating those that might have been biased.

This study, and most like it, defined "added sugar" differently than just "sugar." The latter is almost always sucrose, which you can think of as table sugar. It's what is in those packets labeled "sugar" that you use in your coffee. Sucrose is a disaccharide—a combination of one molecule of glucose (the simplest sugar, and the one in your blood) and one molecule of fructose (fruit sugar).

"Added sugar" can refer to sucrose or any of the other caloric substances we use to sweeten beverages. There are many of these. Some of them are "natural," like honey. Some are extracted from plants but are sugar alcohols, like stevia. Some are syrups made from plants, like agave. Perhaps the most publicized—and demonized—is high-fructose corn syrup, a liquid that contains both glucose and fructose (as does sucrose), but in which those molecules aren't bonded together and just float around separately. Because it's easier to move, cheaper to make, and sweeter than sucrose, high-fructose corn syrup is commonly used in processed foods. But the percentage of fructose (as opposed to glucose) can vary from 42% to 55% depending on what the corn syrup is used for. Remember, sucrose is 50% fructose. Depending on which solution is being used, high-fructose corn syrup isn't necessarily very high in fructose, at least not relative to sucrose.

When people say "added sugar," they're usually talking about all these things. The fructose that occurs naturally in fruit isn't an added sugar, nor is the lactose found in milk (which is a combination of glucose and galactose, another simple sugar). But the sugars we put in foods—including syrups, sucrose, and high-fructose corn syrup—are all added sugars. Compared to the carbs found in unrefined foods—all of which are basically okay for you so long as they're not the only things you're eating—added sugar is pretty much terrible for you unless you severely limit the amount you consume.

For one thing, added sugar has been strongly linked to metabolic diseases such as diabetes. A study published in 2013 used data from the UN's Food and Agriculture Organization to look at the market availability of foods in 175 countries around the world. After controlling for many other factors, the researchers analyzed how the nutritional components of the foods were related to the rates of diabetes in those countries. They found that for every 150 calories of added sugar available each day (about what you'd get in one sugar-sweetened soda), there was a 1.1% increase in the prevalence of type 2 diabetes.

To be fair, these are all epidemiologic studies, and few have the weight of randomized controlled trials. After all, it's hard to imagine anyone being subjected to an increase in added sugar to see if anything bad happens to them, since it's now pretty clear that something will. But even without these trials, the fact remains that large amounts of sugar are not good for you and that removing added sugar from your diet is a good idea.

The larger debate, however, is whether artificial sweeteners are just as bad for you, if not worse, than sugar. As sugar was getting a pass in the 1960s and '70s, the attacks on sugar substitutes were beginning. These attacks didn't just focus on obesity and diabetes, though; they were about something much scarier — cancer.

CAN SACCHARIN AND ASPARTAME GIVE YOU CANCER?

For decades, artificial sweeteners have been condemned as harmful chemicals. Of course, ultimately, everything we eat is a "chemical" of one kind or another. Vitamin C, for instance, is a chemical compound, as are all other vitamins. Just because we call something a chemical doesn't mean it's inherently bad for us. I sometimes wonder whether people who vehemently oppose artificial sweeteners really understand this.

In any case, when it comes to artificial sweeteners, consumers' distrust of chemicals in general has been exacerbated by official warnings about what these particular chemicals might be doing to our health — and especially whether they might be increasing our risk of the dreaded "c word": cancer.

There's some research to back up these cancer warnings. But Diet Coke lovers, take heart: none of it really stands up to scrutiny.

Take saccharin, for example. One of the oldest artificial sweeteners, saccharin was discovered in the late nineteenth century by a German chemist, but it didn't gain widespread popularity until roughly a century later, when it was marketed as a zero-calorie sugar alternative under brand names such as Sweet'N Low. In the 1960s and '70s, consumers in the United States were beginning to feel (fairly enough) that they were consuming too much sugar, and they embraced this sugar substitute. It seemed like a good way to bring down their intake of caloric energy — energy that, if unused, would be converted into fat.

Imagine these dieters' dismay, then, when starting in the 1980s, the U.S. Congress mandated that any product containing saccharin be accompanied by the following warning: "Use of this product may be hazardous to your health. This product contains saccharin, which has been determined to cause cancer in laboratory animals."

I imagine that this kind of language made consumers think twice before using those little packets of sweetener containing saccharin. But what was the basis for Congress's decision?

It turns out that scientists had to work pretty hard to come up with evidence that "determined" a causal link between saccharin and cancer. A summary of the history of saccharin published in the *Annals of Oncology* in 2004 noted that more than fifty studies had been published looking at the use of this sweetener in rats. Twenty of these were one-generation studies, meaning researchers fed rats saccharin and then watched to see what happened. In only one of those studies did huge amounts of saccharin produce cancer, and it was in a type of rat that is frequently infected with a bladder parasite that would leave it susceptible to saccharin-induced bladder cancer.

It seems that some scientists felt that they must be missing something, and they kept going. They started to conduct two-generation studies, in which both the first generation of rats and their offspring were fed lots of saccharin. I imagine the hypothesis was that the saccharin in the parent rats was damaging their DNA or organs in some way that would cause them to pass along a higher risk of cancer to their babies. This sounds somewhat far-fetched to me, but to the scientists' credit, they did indeed find that bladder cancer was significantly more common in the second-generation rats. That prompted many countries in North America and Europe to ban saccharin or attach warnings to it.

I remember those warnings, which came out when I was a kid. Of course, as a child I thought I was immortal and that none of this applied to me. I couldn't believe that I was going to get cancer from something in a packet that I could find on every table in every restaurant. I also thought it was odd that all the warnings specifically noted problems in rats, not people. Ironically, that turned out to be a big deal. This link between saccharin and bladder cancer has never been confirmed in humans. And just because it was observed in rats doesn't mean that other species are likely to demonstrate the same effects. Rats appear to have it especially rough when it comes to bladder cancer.

I'm reminded here of a joke I read once in one of my favorite comic strips, *Bloom County*. It's a zany strip about a town in Middle America that originally ran in U.S. newspapers in the 1980s. (It's now back in an online-only version.) There's this one strip where Opus the penguin, one of the comic's main characters, is rattling off the many things that have been found to cause cancer in rats, to which his young friend Milo replies, "Maybe research causes cancer in rats." I thought this comment was funny at the time, but it turns out there's some truth to it.

Rats, it seems, are more likely to get bladder cancer than humans, especially when you overload them with any number of substances. Feed them large amounts of vitamin C, for instance, and they get bladder cancer. No one has extrapolated this to mean that we should slap labels on orange juice warning people that vitamin C has been determined to cause cancer in laboratory animals.

So rats are more vulnerable to side effects from saccharin than are people, for whom there's no clear evidence of risk. Studies in humans in the UK, Denmark, Canada, and the United States could find no association between saccharin consumption and bladder cancer once the researchers accounted for cigarette smoking (which *does* cause this cancer). Based on these studies, in 2000 saccharin was removed from the carcinogen list maintained by the National Toxicology Program of the United States.

But it was too late. Public perception, once turned against any food, especially a *chemical,* is very hard to change. Removing that warning hasn't made most people I know feel safe. Nor, it turns out, has providing them with other alternatives to sugar.

Aspartame was introduced in the United States in the mid-1970s, around the time saccharin began taking a beating. Early studies showed that aspartame didn't cause cancer in animals, so the scientific and regulatory establishments deemed it safer than saccharin. But in 1996, all that changed when a study titled "Increasing Brain Tumor Rates: Is There a Link to Aspartame?" was published in the *Journal of Neuropathology & Experimental Neurology.*

In journalism, there's an unofficial rule that whenever the title of an article is a question, the answer is "no." But journalists know that if you give an article a title like "Television Won't Literally Rot Your Brain," no one will read it. Title it "Can Television Literally Rot Your Brain?" and it will be all over Facebook.

Intentionally or not, the authors of this study were using this same sleight of hand. While the answer to the question "Is there a link between brain tumors and aspartame?" turned out to be "no" (or at least "not necessarily"), many people (even scientists and doctors) who saw the title ignored the fact that it was a question and jumped to the conclusion that there *was* a connection.

If any of these people had actually bothered to read the report, they would have seen that the authors noted (1) that brain tumors had become more common from 1975 to 1992, and (2) that more people had started consuming aspartame recently. This is correlation, not causation. It tells us about as much as the classic observation that ice cream and murder are both more common when the weather is hot—which is true, but which doesn't mean ice cream causes murder.*

There were other problems with this aspartame–brain tumor logic. The first was that most of the increase in tumors the researchers reported was observed in people age 70 or older, who are not the main consumers of diet soda and aspartame. The second was that the Food and Drug Administration didn't approve aspartame for use until 1981, so blaming it for a rise in tumors in the 1970s was spurious, to say the least. Finally, other, much more comprehensive studies failed to find similar links between aspartame consumption and brain tumors. These include a case-control study of children from the *Journal of the National Cancer Institute* and a cohort study of more than 450,000 adults published in *Cancer Epidemiology, Biomarkers*

---

* This argument, by the way, is similar to the one that links vaccines to autism. Just because the incidence of both these things has gone up simultaneously doesn't mean vaccines cause autism.

& *Prevention*. But neither of these studies had nearly as catchy a title as the first one.

The campaign against aspartame didn't end there. In a 2005 study, scientists claimed that aspartame given to rats caused lymphoma and leukemia, but these conclusions are far from conclusive.* More important, as we saw with saccharin (and in *Bloom County*), there's a big difference between rats and humans.

I don't mean to suggest that aspartame is perfectly safe and can't harm anyone. If you've read chapter 6 on GMOs, you know that it's impossible to say that any foods — including conventionally grown foods — are *completely* safe. This is true for artificial sweeteners, too. For instance, people with phenylketonuria, a rare genetic disorder that makes people hypersensitive to phenylalanine, need to limit their consumption of aspartame, since phenylalanine is one of its components. If they consume too much, they can have seizures or developmental disorders. But for most people, neither aspartame nor saccharin poses any health risks, even if we look beyond cancer.

OTHER MYTHS ABOUT ARTIFICIAL SWEETENERS

There's no widespread conspiracy to hide the "dangers" of artificial sweeteners from you, no matter what that very frightening chain email your mom forwarded you said. That email might have told you how aspartame leads to psychological or behavioral problems, but the studies it cites were either in rats or weren't very well designed. By contrast, a 1998 randomized controlled trial found no neuropsychologic, neurophysiologic, or behavioral issues caused by aspartame. Sure, some people re-

---

* They also saw this relationship only in female rats.

ported symptoms of these problems, but the rates at which they did were similar to those of the people who took a placebo.

I know the chain email told you that aspartame is terrible for kids with ADHD because it exacerbates symptoms or even causes the disorder itself. But another randomized controlled trial, in 1994, showed that even a dose at ten times normal consumption had no effect on children with ADHD. It made no difference in their behavior or in laboratory levels of neurotransmitters, amino acids, or other measures.

But don't take my word for it. A safety review published in *Critical Reviews in Toxicology* in 2007 found that aspartame had been studied extensively and that all the evidence showed it was safe.

Okay, so no cancer and no neurologic effects. But what about diabetes? While I've already discussed the research linking sugar to type 2 diabetes, many health-conscious people are of the opinion that artificial sweeteners can have the same effect. They didn't come to this conclusion on their own. In 2014, a huge study published in *Nature* caused many people to think that artificial sweeteners lead to diabetes. This study also seemed to show that artificial sweeteners can alter the gut microbiome — the ecosystem of bacteria, fungi, and other microscopic organisms that live inside your gut — and that these alterations can lead to diabetes.

When my column on artificial sweeteners appeared in the *New York Times,* this was the study that many angry readers sent to me to show me I was wrong and to prove that these sweeteners are unsafe and harmful. But I hadn't ignored the study; I just didn't think it warranted the huge amount of attention it got.

The researchers described a number of experiments. First, they showed that mice fed aspartame, sucralose (another artificial sweetener), or saccharin had higher blood glucose levels than mice fed water or sugar. Second, they showed that if they sterilized the guts of mice, or cleared out their microbiomes, then transplanted the microbiomes from mice that had been fed artificial sweeteners or sugar into those sterilized mice, the ones that had received transplants from mice fed artificial sweeteners had higher blood glucose levels than those that had received transplants from mice fed sugar. Third, they showed that people who use artificial sweeteners have different levels of enterobacteriaceae, deltaproteobacteria, and actinobacteria in their guts than those who don't. Finally, they looked at five men and two women, all of whom were healthy and didn't use artificial sweeteners. They were given the FDA's maximum allowable amount of saccharin for six days. Four of the seven developed "abnormal glucose responses," and three didn't. The four people who developed the responses also showed changes in the bacteria in their guts.

So what we have here are two studies of mice (again, mice!) that looked at bacteria in their guts over the short term; one relatively small cross-sectional analysis of people's guts that didn't appear to control for anything other than body mass index and that can't establish causality in any case; and a final prospective study of seven people followed for a week. Seven people followed for a week with no control group cannot tell me anything about whether people will get diabetes from saccharin use. I mean, come on. This was a tiny group, and poorly controlled. The cross-sectional study is hard to interpret, too. Maybe people who use artificial sweeteners are different in other ways besides BMI — ways for which the researchers didn't control. Maybe they're different races, they eat different foods, they smoke at different rates, they drink alcohol differently, they're older or younger, and so on. Although I think the results of this study are worthy of follow-up and further research, they don't tell us anything about what artificial sweeteners do to humans in the long run.

There are also a lot of holes in how this study measured the link between artificial sweeteners and metabolic disorders. No one knows how artificial sweeteners affect the bacteria in the gut. No one knows why the three different artificial sweeteners resulted in similar changes when they are completely different molecules. And no one really knows how the interplay between bacteria in the gut affects our health. Some interesting theories purporting to answer all these questions have been proposed, but there is nowhere near any conclusive evidence that artificial sweeteners cause diabetes.

In addition to these unsubstantiated theories about artificial sweeteners causing diabetes, there are arguments out there that artificial sweeteners lead to overweight and obesity. If this is true, it is particularly bad news for the many people who have turned to artificial sweeteners as a way of bringing down their weight. But is it true?

As with the diabetes claim, this one has some basis in research. A study published in the journal *Obesity* in 2008, for instance, looked at how diet beverage consumption was related to weight in more than 3,600 people over the course of seven to eight years. Researchers found that the more diet beverages subjects drank, the higher their risk of being heavier. The media, as you can imagine, covered this finding as *drinking diet beverages may make you gain weight, not lose it.*

This type of research appears again and again. Literally days before I turned in the first draft of this book, another study cropped up; like the aforementioned one, it made headlines. This new study followed more than 1,450 people for about ten years and found that those who consumed low-calorie sweeteners had a higher BMI (a measure of tissue mass used to decide if a person is underweight, normal weight, or overweight), a larger waist circumference, and more abdominal fat than those who didn't consume them.

Studies like these may seem damning — and especially newsworthy because of how bitterly ironic their claims are — but there's a huge problem with them. It's known as *reverse causality* — the tendency of observers to assume that one factor causes another, when it really may be the other way around. For instance, drinking diet soda appears to be associated with being overweight. Haters of diet soda may leap to the conclusion that diet soda causes obesity. But it's also possible that being overweight causes people to drink more diet soda. In fact, that makes a lot of sense. People who are overweight tend to be more likely to diet. People who diet are more likely to drink diet soda.

Reverse causality is often a huge flaw in all kinds of observational studies, and it's a limitation that researchers cannot overcome simply by doing these studies over and over. Observational studies are potentially useful for detecting relationships between things, but they cannot tell us which way the arrow of causality points. Does consuming diet soda make you overweight, or does being overweight make you consume diet soda? Observers — researchers and laypeople alike — often have preconceived notions about which of these causal relationships is true, and start inventing theories as to what might be happening. Some scientists, for instance, hypothesize that people who drink diet soda overcompensate by eating more calories later. Others argue that these beverages change the microbiome and lead to alterations in digestion that cause people to gain weight (or develop diabetes, or what have you). Still others say that the artificial sweeteners in diet soda trick the brain into ordering the body to secrete insulin, which can lead to fat storage and weight gain. Observational studies can't support or refute any of these theories. They just keep reinforcing researchers' beliefs without advancing their knowledge about the causal pathway itself.

If we want to know the real effects of diet soda on weight, we need to look at prospective controlled trials that actually changed the subjects' diets and measured the results. In 2012, for instance, researchers published the results of a trial designed to test whether substituting noncaloric beverages for caloric ones would result in weight loss. It did: people who started drinking diet beverages lost about 2% to 2.5% of their body weight, about the same amount as those who switched to water instead of artificially sweetened beverages. This evidence — that drinking diet soda helps you lose weight — would surely surprise anyone who had made up their mind about artificial sweeteners purely because of those observational studies I mentioned.

When we look at all the studies together, the evidence in favor of artificial sweeteners becomes even more convincing. A meta-analysis published in the *American Journal of Clinical Nutrition* in 2014 examined all of the randomized controlled trials and prospective cohort studies that looked at the relationship between drinking artificially sweetened beverages and body weight. The cohort studies found that diet drinks were significantly associated with a higher BMI. (Remember, these studies just show associations, and reverse causality can be an issue.) But the randomized controlled trials (which are almost always better and can show causality) showed that diet drinks significantly reduced weight, BMI, fat, and waist circumference.

People who want to argue that a food or nutrient is unsafe will often cherry-pick single studies that support their point. This is a common theme in nutrition research. They will always be able to find this kind of ammunition — but not all ammunition is created equal. When people who oppose artificial sweeteners bring up a rat study, I tend to discount it, because artificial sweeteners are easy to study in people, and studies in other species are inherently limited when it comes to drawing conclusions about human health. Even a study of process measures in humans (such as temporary enzyme levels) is worth less than a randomized controlled trial of weight gain or loss. And all of these trials, taken together, offer much more reliable evidence than any single study ever could. When it comes to sugar and artificial sweeteners, the evidence is as strong as can be: the former is much worse for you than the latter.

THE BOTTOM LINE

Some people are convinced that artificial sweeteners are poison. End of story. Nothing that I — let alone the food companies — can say will convince them otherwise. In 2015, Pepsi finally gave up on one such public relations campaign and announced it was going to remove aspartame from Diet Pepsi sold in the United States and replace it with sucralose. Why? Americans were purchasing less Diet Pepsi, and the company had learned through surveys of its customers that the top reason was aspartame. Ironically, the following year Pepsi announced that it was coming out with Diet Pepsi Classic Sweetener Blend, containing — you guessed it — aspartame. Seems that artificial sweetener fans can tell the difference.

As with so many other myths about foods, popular misconceptions about artificial sweeteners are rooted not in logic but in emotion, especially the emotions of fear and disgust. As I said at the beginning of this chapter, of all the things I've admitted publicly, none has earned me as much condemnation as saying that I let my kids drink diet soda. I didn't anticipate — at all — the amount of anger that column would incite. I don't think that letting my children drink diet soda once in a while makes me a monster, but apparently some people do. What blew me away, though, was that people seemed to object to the *diet* even more than to the *soda*.

Even some of my friends appear to have this unscientific bias. Some of them crave sugar-sweetened soda, or even celebrate it as an occasional delicacy. But they can barely contain their disdain when they see my kids drinking Diet Coke.

What's going on here? My children eat a lot of vegetables. They eat a lot of unprocessed foods. They drink a lot of water. Once in a while — not every day, but a few times a week — I let them have diet soda if they wish. Once in a while, I let them have dessert, too. Moderation seems to work, and they're all doing great.

Say all the bad things you want about artificial sweeteners. As far as rigorous research is concerned, the jury is still out on them. The "real" sweetener, sugar, doesn't enjoy the same benefit of the doubt. The epidemiologic evidence suggests correlation — not causation, mind you, but a distinct correlation — between sugar consumption and death, while no such correlation has been detected for artificial sweeteners. In addition, while artificial sweeteners are calorie-free, added sugar is a source of empty calories. Sugar drinks don't fill you up; they just add to your energy intake. How can that be good?

Of course, no one needs soda. Nor does anyone need beer, scotch, cheesesteaks, pizza, or apple pie. But the fact is, I love these things, and I like to have them once in a while. Some people drink nothing but water — more power to them — but most people aren't going to do that. I'm certainly not. Of course, some people overdo it by drinking tons of diet soda, and that *might* not be good for them. (I stress *might*.) Compared to many of the alternatives, though, diet soda seems like a pretty safe choice.

I see a lot of children in my practice who drink gallons of

juice, soda, or milk, and who have a weight problem. The first thing I do is encourage them to eliminate the empty calories of sugar-sweetened beverages. Getting them to switch to water is often very hard. If I can get a child to switch to sugar-free lemonade, at least as a start, it will eliminate hundreds of calories from his or her diet each day.

It's all relative. If I have to choose between diet drinks and those with added sugar, I'll go with the diet. There's a potential — and likely very real — harm from consuming added sugar. There is likely none from artificial sweeteners. In the end, I let my kids drink diet soda because I think it's better than the alternative: soda sweetened with added sugar.

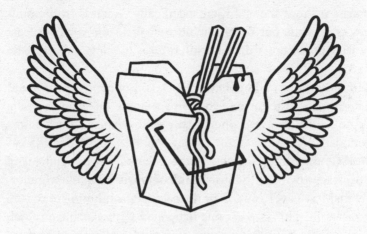

Ten

MSG

THERE'S almost nothing I won't eat. When I met my wife, though, I found that she had a mile-long list of foods she wouldn't touch. This made dining out more difficult than I would have liked. When we lived in Seattle for five years, she wouldn't eat seafood. She missed out on salmon, sushi, and so much more. When we lived in Philadelphia before that, I'm not sure she ate anything besides barbecued chicken or ambiguously "Asian" salads when we went out.

Over time, she's broadened her palate immensely. I depend on her now to find the interesting restaurants in town, and I'm amazed at how she is drawn specifically to foods from countries other than our own. There's very little she won't at least try. But there's one thing she still refuses to allow on her plate: MSG.

Monosodium glutamate, or MSG, is a chemical compound that enhances the taste of food. It's a staple of Asian cooking. It's delicious. It's also one of the most despised ingredients around.

MSG sometimes seems to have become more a subject of conspiracy theories than of health science. People are generally suspicious of it, and their distrust seems immune to reason or research. This is what has happened with vaccines (which many people now think cause autism); it's what's happening with artificial sweeteners (which, as I explained in the last chapter, are blamed for cancer, obesity, diabetes, and more). But when it comes to MSG, the arguments against it are downright bizarre.

If you don't believe me, go to any Internet search engine and type in "MSG." Pair that search term with the name of a widespread health issue. It doesn't matter what you pick — autism, obesity, Alzheimer's, ADHD. Any number of links to websites claiming that MSG somehow contributes to that problem will pop up.

As with other medical conspiracy theories, the ones regarding MSG may be impossible to disprove or dispel. We've seen this with the myth about the connection between vaccines and autism. This supposed link came out of a case series published in the prestigious medical journal the *Lancet*. This study had a lot of flaws, and it was later retracted by the journal (a rare occurrence). A later investigation found that a number of the children described in the study didn't have autism, and many had symptoms before receiving vaccines. Dates had been changed, as had laboratory results, and the study had been commissioned and funded by a group planning litigation against vaccine manufacturers. The editors at the *BMJ* called the whole thing a "fraud." None of that had any effect. Once the genie was out of the bottle, it didn't matter how much research refuted the original claim. Fear had settled into the public consciousness, and it became almost counterproductive to try to set the record straight.

MSG is still used by the food industry in lots of processed foods — and, of course, in Asian food. But companies try to be subtle about it because they know that consumers are wary. Many of the products that contain it are those we consider unhealthy. Because we associate MSG with them, we continue to believe that it's unhealthy, too. But it's not; it's delicious. What's more, without its key ingredient — an organic compound called glutamate — you wouldn't be alive to read these words.

Unfortunately, too few people acknowledge the role this "chemical" in MSG plays in our bodies. Indeed, many stop listening to all the reassuring evidence about MSG as soon as they hear the word "chemical." But just because glutamate is a chemical doesn't mean it's bad for you. After all, which of the foods we eat *aren't* chemicals?

COME ON, PEOPLE — *EVERYTHING* IS A CHEMICAL

Everything we consume, even water, is a chemical. That word alone shouldn't scare us away from MSG. Nor should the claim that it's "unnatural." Plenty of *real* toxins, like botulinum (the protein that causes the disease botulism), are natural,* and I wouldn't advocate eating any of those.

Not everyone shares this nuanced view of chemicals. A number of personalities in the nutrition world have made quite a name for themselves (and a lot of money) by attacking food chains and producers for using chemicals in their food. One of the better known is Vani Hari, "the Food Babe."

Not long ago, Hari went after companies for including the additive carrageenan in their products. Carrageenan is used to help foods thicken or gel. It's as good an example as any for understanding the process by which people attack chemicals in food. Their condemnations tend to follow a certain pattern.

First, in August 2014 Hari provided a link to a report citing animal studies in which mice and other animals given huge quantities of carrageenan developed a host of problems, including intestinal lesions and cancer. As I've shown throughout this book, just because something is true for animals doesn't mean it's true for humans. But you wouldn't know that to hear Hari tell it.

What's more, Hari cited stories of human studies showing that people who ate carrageenan were more likely to have a host of disorders, including diabetes and irritable bowel syndrome. Yet she made no reference to the fact that these studies were almost always case-control or retrospective cohort studies. As I've noted elsewhere in this book, those kinds of studies suffer from certain biases and, like observational (as opposed to experimental) studies, are capable of proving only correlation, not causation. Hari also pointed to the fact that the World Health Organization and National Research Council have labeled carrageenan a carcinogen. As we saw in the chapters on meat and

---

* What else? Tetanus, diphtheria, methylmercury, cyanide, arsenic, belladonna . . . I could do this all day.

coffee, however, the WHO has labeled almost anything you can think of as potentially causing cancer. Tellingly, the organization gave carrageenan a 2B rating, for "possibly carcinogenic," a category shared by pickles, and — until recently — coffee.

If Hari's plan of attack sounds familiar, it's because it's similar to the way other members of the science and nutrition establishments have gone after other supposedly "bad" foods such as artificial sweeteners and meat. It's a tried-and-true method of scaring people into giving up certain foods.

Another well-publicized example in the war against chemicals in food, and one that also features Vani Hari, came in 2014 when anti-chemical crusaders directed their wrath at Subway sandwiches. It turns out that Subway's bread contained azodicarbonamide, which works as both a flour bleaching agent and a dough conditioner. In other words, it helps make bread appear whiter and have a better texture.

But azodicarbonamide has other uses as well. When heated, it breaks down and releases nitrogen, carbon dioxide, and other gases. When it's incorporated into a variety of products, therefore, it can result in the formation of bubbles, yielding springier, bouncier substances. If you add it to vinyl foam, for instance, you can use the foam to make yoga mats.

As one might expect, Hari and other anti-chemical zealots zeroed in on this application of azodicarbonamide in their attacks on Subway. They argued that when you eat Subway sandwiches, you're basically eating yoga mats. Who would want to do that?

Many organizations have determined that low levels of azodicarbonamide, especially those used in foods, are safe. But this didn't matter to the crusaders. It's a chemical; it had to go. After Subway caved in and removed it, many other fast-food chains followed suit. None of them wanted the bad publicity of making their rolls or breads out of yoga mats.

Just because we can use a substance for industrial purposes doesn't mean it can't also be eaten as food. Corn can be used to create ethanol, for instance, which can be added to gasoline to help power our cars. That doesn't mean corn is dangerous, or that every time you enjoy an ear of corn you're eating gasoline. To take another example, I've read a number of articles in recent years that talk about promising research into turning glucose into diesel fuel or polyester. But that doesn't mean that when you consume glucose, you're eating pants. Any chemical — or any other substance, for that matter — can have more than one use.

In the case of MSG, our collective inability to reckon with this fact is especially frustrating, because MSG — or at least its key chemical compound — is quite literally the stuff of life.

THE REAL STUFF OF LIFE

Human beings can recognize five basic tastes. We evolved to perceive them so we'd be able to tell which foods are good for us and which might be harmful. Sweet foods encourage us to get carbohydrates into our bodies so that we have enough energy to live. Salty foods encourage us to ingest enough sodium to maintain the body's water balance. Sour tastes can be good or bad, helping us to figure out when food is okay to eat (ripe) and when it's not (spoiled). Bitter tastes, for the most part, are warnings that something isn't good for us, and maybe even poisonous. The fifth taste, and the most widely misunderstood, is umami.

The word "umami" comes from the Japanese word meaning "delicious flavor." This earthy, rich taste is distinctive in meat broths, fish sauces, and a number of fermented products. We likely developed the ability to sense umami to help ensure that we would eat enough protein. The taste of MSG alone is rather odd — it's sort of salty and sort of meaty — but when combined with other tastes, it can be magical.

The receptors on the tongue that respond to umami are the ones that recognize glutamate, one of the amino acids (more on those in a minute) that make up all proteins in the human body. Glutamate is also found in tomatoes, cheese, and many seaweeds. When we add one sodium (salt) molecule to glutamate, we get monosodium glutamate, or MSG.

That's right. Contrary to what you may have thought, the crucial building block of MSG is a naturally occurring substance, glutamate, not something that was created in some mad scientist's lab. Not only that, but glutamate is essential to our survival.

I'm going to get a little wonky here, but this is a perfect — and important — example of how a chemical can unfairly get a bad rap. So bear with me while I explain how the amino acid that is the crux of MSG is also crucial to our very existence.

All human life is encoded in our DNA by four molecules known as nucleotides: adenine (A), guanine (G), cytosine (C), and thymine (T). These four molecules are put together in groups of three known as codons. These codons are ordered in such a way as to spell out the code for building everything in our bodies, mostly through proteins.

Codons — or the three-letter groupings representing them — are code words for amino acids, which are the building blocks of proteins. Only twenty of them are used in the human body, and every single protein that we need or use is created from them. Nine of the amino acids are called "essential" because we can't make them on our own; we need to eat them in order to survive. The other eleven amino acids can be produced internally, but that doesn't make them any less important. One of these internally produced amino acids is glutamic acid. Glutamate is glutamic acid that's lost a hydrogen atom. The two substances are basically interchangeable.

Glutamic acid, like some other amino acids, is more than just a component of larger proteins. It is, for instance, a key part of the mechanism by which cells create energy; without this mechanism, all oxygen-dependent life as we know it would die. Glutamic acid is also one of the main players in how the body gets rid of waste through urea. Glutamate is even one of the key neurotransmitters used by the neurons in our brains to pass messages.

Without glutamate, we would not be able to think or pee, and we would die. This chemical, in short, is absolutely, positively essential to our survival. So anyone who tells you that the "stuff" in MSG is bad for you is deluding themselves — or maybe just short on glutamate.

Anyway, the joke's on them. Even the most ardent haters of MSG are consuming glutamic acid every day. That's because it's in all proteins, even the ones we eat. When the body breaks down those proteins through digestion, it provides us with much of our supply of glutamic acid. Some foods also contain "free" glutamic acid — the kind we don't have to break down proteins to get. Fermentation, for instance, results in an increased amount of free glutamic acid in foods. Some foods produce free glutamic acid naturally, and it was from one of those foods that glutamic acid was first isolated, in 1908.

It turns out that certain seaweeds common in Japanese cooking contain a ton of free glutamic acid. But in 1908, when a scientist named Kikunae Ikeda managed to extract glutamic acid from seaweed, he was left with a liquid mess that couldn't be easily packaged. To stabilize it, he combined it with salt to make a solid. That was the invention of monosodium glutamate — MSG.

Today, we can make MSG even more easily than Ikeda did.

The bacterium *Corynebacterium glutamicum* produces pure glutamic acid as waste when it consumes glucose (or sugar) from any number of vegetable sources. Yes, this is done in a lab to produce MSG, but the underlying process is completely "natural." After these bacteria work their magic, scientists filter off the glutamic acid, purify it, add sodium to make it crystallize, and ta-da: we have good old-fashioned MSG.

It took a while, but within the next decade, scientists had figured out how to mass-produce MSG. Just as the use of glutamate-containing foods was widely popular in Asia, the use of MSG (which is packaged like salt) blossomed there as well. But the inherent appeal of MSG, or rather of the basic taste it creates, was and is by no means limited to Asia. Go into a trendy restaurant in any Western city these days, and you'll likely hear about the importance of umami from your server or a fellow diner. There's even a restaurant in New York City called Umami Burger. The umami in this restaurant's burgers often comes from "natural" glutamate — that is, from ingredients that contain relatively large amounts of this chemical. The glutamate in those ingredients is exactly the same thing as the glutamate in MSG.

But don't try telling the upscale diners at Umami Burger that their expensive, "all-natural" burgers are basically giving them the same effect — and the same amino acids — as MSG. That ship has long since sailed.

CHINESE RESTAURANT SYNDROME

Although MSG became a staple in Asia rather quickly, it took longer for it to reach the shores of America. Only in the 1950s, some forty years after it was first commercially produced on the other side of the Pacific, did it begin to make its way into

processed foods in the United States. It wasn't just in the unhealthy stuff either. MSG was added to canned vegetables, tomato sauce, soup, and more. It even started to appear in baby
food. What the babies thought of it, we'll never know, but
American cooks and consumers seemed to appreciate the taste
it added to their dishes. Dig up some recipes from around this
time, and odds are at least one of them will call for MSG.

But a reckoning was coming. It's possible that the growing
concerns about artificial sweeteners, and the federal bans that
resulted from the (mistaken) belief that they caused cancer (see
chapter 9), led to a backlash against "chemicals" in our food.
MSG may have gotten caught up in this hysteria.

In 1968, a doctor and senior research investigator at the National Biomedical Research Foundation published a short letter in the *New England Journal of Medicine* titled "Chinese-Restaurant Syndrome." He described how, in the years since he'd
moved to the United States from China, he'd noticed that he
had some symptoms that came on about fifteen to twenty min-
utes after he ate at a Chinese restaurant, especially restaurants
that served "Northern Chinese food," as he called it. The symptoms included numbness on the back of his neck, spreading to
his arms and back; weakness; and palpitations. He didn't necessarily blame these troubles on MSG, but asked if anyone else
noticed these issues.

Evidently, this doctor wasn't alone. The *New England Journal of Medicine* was flooded with responses. The next month,
the *New York Times* joined the fray with an article headlined
"Chinese Restaurant Syndrome Puzzles Doctors." If you read
the article, you'll see that it's written by a skeptical physician.
But, as often seems to happen, the publicity reinforced beliefs
about the dangers of MSG even as many articles sought to question those beliefs. In fact, many who reference the *New York*

Times article today use it to support the claims about Chinese restaurant syndrome. There are also many who believe that Chinese restaurant syndrome — which, in a headline roughly a decade later, the *New York Times* called "That Won-Ton Soup Headache" (I wish I was making this up) — was somewhat based in racism and a mistrust of the "exotic" in America in the late 1960s and 1970s.

Whatever the cause, the initial flurry of attention in the late 1960s led to further studies, which only fueled speculation about the health risks of MSG. In 1969, one year after the letter appeared in the *New England Journal of Medicine,* a study published in *Science* explored how MSG affected mice. The researcher reported that mice injected with MSG developed necrotic brain lesions and neuroendocrine disorders and also became obese.

All it takes is a little bit of science, a couple of impaired mice, and a few news stories to make people lose their minds about a given food. As it was with artificial sweeteners, so it was with MSG. It didn't matter that the MSG in the 1969 study was injected under the skin of mice instead of being eaten (which is how we get it into our bodies). It didn't matter that the amount of MSG administered in the trial would be more appropriate for an elephant than a mouse. (As recently as 2002, researchers were feeding 20 grams of MSG a day to rats for up to six months to show that it hurt their eyes. Humans don't eat anywhere near that much; the average amount an American consumes is about half a gram a day, and the most we consume in a meal is a few grams.) And it didn't matter that MSG had been in human foods for a long time without demonstrating any adverse effects like the ones these researchers observed in their rodent subjects. Anecdotes — the lowliest of all forms of scientific evidence — fueled the fire. Lorne Greene, the famous star of TV's

Bonanza, was hospitalized for four days because he fainted after eating at a Chinese restaurant, and everyone just *knew* why. MSG was poison, and we needed to get rid of it.

And get rid of MSG we did. Nutrition experts, along with advocates such as Ralph Nader, went to Congress to argue that MSG had to come out of baby food. After all, did we really want to poison our children? In late 1969, most of the baby food producers gave up and voluntarily pulled MSG from their products. This, of course, only reinforced the idea that MSG was unsafe and needed to be removed from more foods. Unlike other ingredients (such as artificial sweeteners), however, the Food and Drug Administration never ruled that MSG wasn't "generally recognized as safe." Companies got rid of it voluntarily.

Interestingly, at no point during this push and pull did anyone seem to acknowledge that human milk contains considerable glutamate and glutamic acid — more than baby formula and cow's milk. Scientists have hypothesized that human milk's relatively high level of glutamate is the result of an adaptation, one that helped ensure that babies will drink enough nourishing milk — because it tastes so good to them. Yet no one suggested that we ban breast milk because it contains the same substance as that controversial baby food.

What's amazing about all of this is that people immediately jumped from Chinese restaurant syndrome to MSG without considering that it might be something else in the food that was at work. After all, Chinese cooking uses a set of ingredients that is different from that of other cultures. There's no reason to believe that some people — like the doctor who gave Chinese restaurant syndrome its name — couldn't be sensitive or allergic to those.

Chinese food, for instance, sometimes contains rather high levels of histamine, which is found in shrimp, tofu, and many sauces. Histamine, of course, is the substance in the body that can lead to allergic reactions. When Chinese food contains a lot of it, it can essentially have the opposite effect as drugs like Benadryl. These "antihistamines" block the histamine pathway, helping to alleviate allergy symptoms. By contrast, foods high in histamine can cause the body to release histamine. It's not inconceivable that some foods like this could cause allergy-like symptoms.

This alternative narrative about Chinese restaurant syndrome didn't factor into the conversation about MSG at all, nor did it stem the growing tide of "evidence" about its unhealthiness. Over the next few decades, researchers killed innumerable animals trying to prove that MSG was horrible for human beings. If you search for it, you will find research showing that huge amounts of MSG given to small animals produced bad outcomes. You will also find case reports, and even case-control studies, arguing that MSG consumption is associated with disease and disability in humans. But good research — the only kind we should pay attention to when determining our own diets — tells a different story.

MSG WILL NOT HURT YOU

We can kill rats with huge doses of a particular food, but that proves nothing about what the food does to humans when consumed as part of a typical diet. It takes careful thinking and planning, and the use of human subjects consuming normal amounts of the food, to prove what effects the food does or does not have on us.

Experimental research into MSG has revealed that it has few, if any, effects on humans. For instance, in a 1993 study published in the journal *Food and Chemical Toxicology*, researchers gave seventy-one healthy people a randomized dose of either 0 (placebo), 1.5, 3, or 3.15 grams of MSG. The researchers worked hard to make sure the participants couldn't tell what they were ingesting. About 15% of those who ingested MSG reported sensations of some sort. But so did 14% of the people who consumed the placebo. The differences weren't significant. (In fact, these researchers found that a lot of the prior research was likely biased, because in the high doses used in studies, MSG tastes really bad. And when you feed people stuff that tastes bad, they are more likely to report bad things.)

A few years later, another experiment debunked the myth that people with asthma might put themselves at higher risk of an asthma attack from eating MSG. This study, the results of which were published in 1998, followed twelve people with asthma after they consumed no MSG, 1 or 5 grams of MSG, or a placebo. The researchers detected no MSG-induced asthma effects.

To be sure, that was a small study, but a larger trial reached the same conclusion. In 1999, the *Journal of Allergy and Clinical Immunology* published the results of a randomized controlled trial of one hundred people who had asthma. Thirty of them had a history of Chinese restaurant syndrome, and seventy did not. They were all given 2.5 grams of MSG (a hefty dose, considering that the average American consumes about half a gram of MSG a day). Consuming this large amount of MSG produced no additional asthma symptoms in either group, even in subjects who thought they were sensitive to MSG compared with those who did not.

Some scientists and consumer advocates remained unconvinced. They argued that a subset of people still existed for whom MSG was bad, and that studies failed to include this specific population. So in 2000, researchers published a study so thorough that it should have ended any controversy over MSG.

These researchers assembled a group of 130 people who all

said they suffered from a sensitivity to MSG. The researchers gave them, on separate days, either 5 mg of MSG or 5 mg of a placebo. They then asked the people to report how many symptoms they felt (out of a list of ten). About two-thirds of the subjects reported at least two symptoms on both days.

The researchers asked those people to repeat the study, and seventy-six did. Only nineteen of them reported at least two symptoms when consuming 5 mg of MSG but not when consuming the placebo. Remember, all of these people said they were sensitive to MSG when the study began.

These nineteen people were then asked to go through the cycle two more times, and twelve accepted. Only two of them repeatedly showed at least two symptoms with MSG and none with the placebo. The symptoms were inconsistent, however, which left open the possibility that something besides MSG was at work here.

But the researchers *still* weren't done. They asked the only two subjects who had consistently responded to MSG and not to the placebo to repeat the trial three more times. Both of them responded to only one of the three MSG challenges. They didn't have any symptoms the other two times.

In other words, even when given huge doses of MSG — about ten times what the average person eats in a day, way more than what they'd get in any one meal — the subjects of this study didn't have any consistent reactions to the substance, if they had any reaction at all.

THE BOTTOM LINE

Glutamate isn't just delicious; it's necessary for your survival. You don't need to eat MSG to get glutamate, but there's no good evidence that it's going to hurt you. So why deprive yourself?

I play in a weekly gaming group.* In addition to beer, some of the participants bring snacks to the meeting for everyone to enjoy. Many of these snacks are purchased at international markets. Sometimes the snacks taste just terrible. But other times they're mind-blowingly good — often thanks to their MSG content.

Recently, we broke into some bags of Takis, which are made by a Mexican company. Takis are rolled-up tortilla chips, sort of like tube-shaped Doritos. The taste of these MSG-laden snacks is hard to describe. When you bite into them, you're hit with an almost overwhelming burst of umami — one so utterly delicious that you immediately want to eat more. The taste lingers afterward, too. Just writing about them, I'm salivating.

My point is that people in other countries don't seem to eschew MSG the way we do in the United States. MSG is ubiquitous in the cuisines of Japan, China, and many other Asian countries. It's in these snacks from Mexico. There's no evidence that people in those countries suffer disproportionately from headaches, asthma, or other afflictions that more-MSG-averse cultures commonly associate with this ingredient. If the people who eat the most MSG have no fear of it, why should we?

---

* Yes, I still play Dungeons & Dragons. My sons play, too. They don't get to drink the beer.

NON-ORGANIC FOODS

WHEN I was a kid growing up in Philadelphia, seeing a goat or a chicken meant that I was on some sort of field trip. Once I moved to Indiana, sights like this became part of my commute. Seriously. When I left my house each morning, I was almost immediately confronted by a fenced-in yard full of goats, chickens, and one cow. It wasn't a farm either, just someone's home.

There are perks to living really close to farmland, and one of them is that you have much better access to farmers' markets, and the fresh produce and foods they have to offer. Soon after moving to Indiana, my family purchased a "farm share," and each week we would go to a central location and pick up a box of organically grown fruits, vegetables, and eggs. It would be fair to say that this completely changed our eating habits. We started eating a wider variety of vegetables, prepared in new ways. Our consumption of pasta and bread, even of meat, went down. My wife became much more aware of how the foods we were eating were produced, with the effect that we started eating more unprocessed and humanely raised foods.

Slowly, however, other standards starting creeping in. Before long, everything that passed our family's lips had to be "organic." Aimee argued that organic foods were better for us. She thought they were more nutritious. She even seemed to believe they were safer to eat than conventionally grown foods.

When this started, she applied this standard only to fruits, vegetables, and eggs. The stuff we were eating was so good that I didn't care to argue. But soon her obsession went beyond what we were buying directly from the local farm. She began to look for the organic label on everything. She even began to buy organic cane sugar.

This shift to organic foods made the scientist in me uncomfortable. After all, organic cane sugar is considerably more expensive than regular cane sugar, but it's still just molecules of sucrose, right? I mean, what else could it be?

I like being married, so I let it go for a time. But when we had an argument at Thanksgiving because she refused to eat non-organic gravy for the turkey, I'd had enough. I felt compelled to look at the evidence to see whether the things she believed were true. What I found surprised both of us, and affected our household in a pretty fundamental way. Our marriage clearly survived—but our all-organic meal plan did not.

WHAT MAKES A FOOD "ORGANIC"?

Given how much I hear the word "organic," I assumed there must be a simple definition of this term. When I went to the USDA website, however, I learned that this is far from the truth. This seemingly simple term is actually wildly compli-cated to define.*

Here's the best I can do without taking up too much space in this book. According to the USDA, organic crops can't have any prohibited substances (meaning most synthetic pesticides, herbicides, and fertilizers) applied to the land on which they're grown for at least three years before they're planted. Fertilizers have to be either non-synthetic or an allowable synthetic mate-rial; herbicides and pesticides need to be natural or on the ap-proved synthetic list. Seeds need to be organic, and no mucking with the genes. Starting in the last third of gestation, livestock must be fed only organic feed, although some vitamin and min-eral supplements are allowed. Dairy livestock need to be or-ganically raised for a year before the milk can be considered organic. Sick animals can be treated only with approved sub-stances. Ruminants have to be pastured for at least 120 days of the grazing season and get at least 30% of their feed from pas-ture. All animals need access to the outdoors year-round. The USDA has additional handling standards and regulations for labeling multi-ingredient products. For an item to be labeled

---

* There's a monster list of terms related to the USDA's National Organic Program. You have to see it to believe it: https://goo.gl/W6XhSO.

"certified organic," the agency requires that at least 95% of its ingredients be organic. The other 5% can be pretty much anything. (Nothing's perfect.)*

A hundred years ago, "organic" meant exactly what our current mythology holds it to mean. Consumers were confident that their food was produced locally, by small farmers who did not use pesticides, herbicides, antibiotics, synthetic fertilizers, or genetic manipulation when growing fruits and vegetables or raising animals. That's because these technologies simply did not exist at the time.

Today, even foods labeled "organic" can contain non-organic ingredients, yet the mystique around the term has given rise to a hugely profitable business for food companies. It's responsible for more than $31 billion in sales each year in the United States. More than 4% of the food items sold in this country are organic, and gigantic companies have cropped up solely to promote and sell them. In many ways, organic foods are now every bit as corporate as the conventionally grown stuff, with bucolic brands and packages obscuring the gears of the industrial food system. "Cascadian Farm" is owned by General Mills. "Back to Nature" was owned for some time by Kraft, which in 2012 sold it to Brynwood Partners, a private equity fund. "MorningStar Farms" is owned by Kellogg.

One of the advantages of this commercialization — if you're open to such lines of thought — is that it has driven down the cost of organic foods, which is higher than that of conventionally grown foods. I'm not just talking about the difference in price you see between a market like Whole Foods and cheaper supermarket chains. All organic foods cost more than conven-

---

* It may seem that I'm being dismissive of the USDA's "certified organic" label, but at least the agency has some standards and verification, even if the verification process is weak. Many other labels mean even less. "Antibiotic-free," "free-range," "hormone-free," and "natural," for example, are vague and have no standard definitions.

tional foods. In 2016, the USDA's Economic Research Service released data on the price differences for seventeen types of foods. On the low end, organic spinach cost 7% more, organic granola 22% more, and organic carrots, potatoes, and apples 27% to 29% more. Organic baby food, popular among so many moms, cost about 30% more on average. But that's by no means the biggest markup. Organic salad mix costs 60% more than conventionally grown salad mix. Organic milk costs 72% more. Organic eggs cost 82% more.

Why are organic foods so much more expensive? It's not necessarily because organic farmers and big food companies are greedy. Rather, it's largely because organic foods cost more to produce. Organic growers need to jump through lots of hoops to get their pesticides, farming methods, and foods certified. Since the organic certification of animal products (milk and eggs) requires extra time and effort, the premium paid for those products is higher than it is for organic produce.

The good news is that the price difference between organic foods and non-organic foods has been dropping over time. For some organic foods, the premium is now less than it used to be, but that's not true for all of them. And for some foods (again, milk and eggs), the premium has actually been rising in recent years. Why? I'm not sure.

Higher prices haven't dissuaded people from buying more and more organic foods. In 2004, about 5% of the spinach consumers bought was organically grown. By 2010, that percentage had increased to 40%, meaning that the share of people eating conventionally grown spinach dropped from 95% to 60% in just six years.

The mainstreaming of organic foods is relatively recent; the USDA didn't create regulations for organic foods until 2002. Despite their relative novelty and spreading roots in the industrial food system, many people agree with my wife that organic foods are healthier than non-organic ones, and consumers are willing to pay more for them. But are they right?

ORGANIC FOODS ARE NO BETTER FOR YOU THAN CONVENTIONALLY GROWN FOODS

When it comes to dietary health, there's little evidence that organic foods are superior to the non-organic variety.

The most thorough study I've seen on this topic was published in 2012 in the *Annals of Internal Medicine*. Researchers at Stanford University conducted a systematic review of all the research published in the medical literature between 1996 and 2009 that compared organic and conventionally grown foods.

A total of 223 studies compared the nutritional content and contaminants (such as bacteria, pesticides, fungi, and heavy metals) in foods grown organically and foods grown conventionally. One hundred fifty-three of these studies looked at fruits, vegetables, and grains; seventy-one looked at meat, poultry, and eggs; some overlapped. On both of these metrics — nutritional content and contaminants — the Stanford researchers found no meaningful differences between organic and non-organic foods.

On the nutritional front, the researchers detected no significant differences in vitamin content. Of the eleven other nutrients they looked at (potassium, calcium, phosphorus, magnesium, iron, protein, fiber, quercetin, kaempferol, flavanols, and phenols), they detected statistically significant differences in only two: phosphorus (due to a single, outlying study) and phenols (due mostly to two studies that were also outliers and that did not report sample size, which is really odd).

When researchers conduct studies over and over again, we

hope the results will cluster around some value that we can comfortably view as "right." An outlier is a study whose results are far from that central value. If we do ten studies looking at the weight of mice, and in nine of them the weight ranges from 0.7 to 1.3 pounds but the tenth reports 25 pounds, that study is an outlier. Outliers tend to be less trustworthy than studies that are close to the central value, and sometimes they're simply wrong. In a meta-analysis, however, one outlier can really change the results of the study, since it can drag the final average result away from the true average.

Sample sizes need to be calculated so that we are confident we have enough subjects to know the results can be believed. It's a part of good science. A study that lacks such a calculation should, perhaps, be viewed with more skepticism. The two phenol studies mentioned earlier not only didn't have this important calculation, but they were outliers — making them doubly concerning. If the results of these studies are discounted, the overall conclusion is that there was no difference between organic and non-organic plant and animal products with respect to nutrients.

When the Stanford researchers looked at the nutritional content of organic versus non-organic milk, they found that some studies reported that organic milk had more omega-3 fatty acids than conventional milk. But most of these studies were looking at raw milk, which represents only a fraction of the milk consumed in Europe and practically none of it consumed in North America. (Besides which, why are people drinking so much milk anyway? Haven't they seen the research presented in chapter 1?)

As with nutritional content, the *Annals of Internal Medicine* meta-analysis did not reveal much of a difference in contaminant levels between organic and non-organic foods. When the researchers looked at pesticide levels, they found that organic foods *did* have a significantly lower chance of being free of any pesticides at all, which isn't surprising given that hardly any synthetic pesticides are allowed to be used in growing certified organic foods. But the levels of pesticides detected in nonorganic foods were under the maximum allowed safety limits, so this difference was actually not all that clinically significant. There was even less of a disparity between the two types of foods when it came to other contaminants. Bacterial contamination with E. coli, for instance, was found in 7% of organic foods and 6% of conventionally grown foods—no significant difference. The same was true for other bacteria, fungi, and heavy metals.

Although measuring nutrients and contaminants is all well and good, what we really care about is what happens to actual people who eat this stuff. Are they healthier? The Stanford researchers looked at this, too, and found no meaningful difference there either.

To assess the effects of organic and conventional foods on human health, these researchers analyzed studies of fourteen different populations. These studies included more than 13,800 participants. Two of them looked at children and pregnant women to see if the type of foods they ate (either organic or non-organic) affected whether they developed asthma, eczema, wheezing, or other symptoms or markers of atopic disease; it didn't. Eleven more looked at men and non-pregnant women, mostly examining biomarker levels of certain health factors in the serum, urine, breast milk, and semen of those who ate either organic or conventionally grown foods; overall, there was no significant difference. Only one of the studies looked at clinical outcomes, but it found that eating organic meat in the winter actually increased the risk of illness due to campylobacter infection—a result that is hard to explain and is certainly not conclusive, though it is likely not the result that many organic acolytes would expect.

In the world of epidemiology, 223 studies constitute an enormous body of research. And if this sort of rigorous science failed to reveal any real health benefits or protections from eating organic foods, that's enough to convince me to withhold judgment about the conventional stuff — even in the face of lesser evidence that argues the opposite.

Not long after the *Annals of Internal Medicine* meta-analysis was published, a newer study in the *British Journal of Nutrition* seemed to refute it, finding that organic fruits and vegetables were more nutritious and safer than non-organic ones. Its authors declared it to be the "most extensive analysis" of its kind. Organic believers said that it trumped all other studies and should be declared the final word.

The authors of this study, a group of scientists from all over the world, claimed that the existing research into the health effects of organic and non-organic foods wasn't "comprehensive" enough. They combed the literature from 1992 through 2011, which overlaps with the Stanford researchers' work, and ultimately reviewed 448 studies. They decided that 343 of them were appropriate for inclusion. Using this larger, less rigorously selected body of evidence, they declared that organic foods are safer and more nutritious than conventional foods. Pretty much the only evidence they had for this claim was their finding that organic foods contain significantly higher levels of antioxidants than conventionally grown foods, as well as lower levels of synthetic pesticides.

There are a couple of problems with this logic. For one thing, concerns about higher levels of pesticides in non-organic foods were addressed in the *Annals of Internal Medicine* study, which reported that none of the studies these researchers analyzed had detected levels of synthetic pesticides that came anywhere near what is generally recognized to be unsafe. But perhaps the bigger issue is that antioxidant content simply isn't the way we decide whether a food is nutritious.

Antioxidants are chemical compounds that our bodies use to combat "free radicals," another type of compound. Free radicals harm us by stealing electrons from molecules, which can damage structures in cells, including DNA. Depending on which molecules are damaged and how they are damaged, free radicals can even lead to cancer. Antioxidants protect us by "giving" electrons to free radicals so they won't take them from our cells.

But antioxidants vary a great deal in makeup, and different antioxidants work in different ways in different parts of the body. Vitamins C and E are both antioxidants, but the former is water-soluble and prevents scurvy, while the latter is fat-soluble and helps protect cell membranes. What's more, there's little evidence, if any, that consuming extra antioxidants can measurably improve our health. Various studies on vitamin E, for instance, have yielded mixed results about its role in improving health. Other studies focusing on beta-carotene, another antioxidant, have shown that it has no effect in preventing heart disease or cancer. Yet more studies looking at mixtures of antioxidants have found that they, too, don't prevent cardiovascular events in women, or cancer, heart disease, or death in women or men.

All of these studies involved much higher doses of antioxidants than you could possibly get by eating organic foods. So it stands to reason that if the studies' massive supplementation of antioxidants had no effect on participants' health, eating organic foods would have no effect on the average consumer either.

When a newer systematic review is less rigorous than a previous study in judging the quality of the research it includes, we should be wary of any benefit it reports. It's entirely possible, of course, that previous researchers might have made mistakes and missed important studies, but that doesn't seem to be the case here. The newer *British Journal of Nutrition* study looked at more studies than the *Annals of Internal Medicine* study did, but only by including research that was of lower methodological quality. In my mind, that's not a selling point. Even if you don't see that as a problem, you can't ignore the fact that the differences the *British Journal of Nutrition* study found between organic and non-organic foods, though statistically significant, make no real difference in terms of actual nutrition or safety. The facts that conventionally grown foods have a lesser amount of antioxidants and contain some, though not unsafe levels of, pesticides does not prove that they are unhealthy.

There's one more reason to prefer the *Annals of Internal Medicine* study to the *British Journal of Nutrition* one. The former was apparently done with no external funding, while the latter, which cost $429,000, was funded by a charity that "supports organic farming research."* I'm not saying that this potential conflict of interest tainted the study, but it should at least be acknowledged that such a conflict exists when weighing the two studies against each other.

Not enough attention is paid to issues like these, or to assessments that don't fit the dominant, tidy narrative about studies in the popular press. For instance, although few news stories reported it, the *British Journal of Nutrition* study found that organic crops are significantly lower in protein than conventionally grown crops. Protein is an actual nutrient, unlike antioxidants, and if organic foods might actually contain less of it, that

---

* For the record, $429,000 is a massive amount of money for a systematic review. I don't know of any other review that has come close to this.

is something we need to look into further. But this sort of nuance tends to get lost in the translation.

Oversimplification isn't surprising in a black-and-white comparison like the one between organic and non-organic foods. It should, however, make us rethink the importance we place on these categories in the first place.

IT'S TIME FOR A NEW PARADIGM

Not only is the organic versus non-organic debate based on a flimsy distinction between these two categories, but the choices it gives us are also suboptimal.

Consider the other reasons people turn to organic foods, apart from their ostensibly superior nutritional content and lower levels of contaminants. Besides organic foods' effect on our health, one of the big reasons people cite for buying them is that organic farming is better for the environment because it uses fewer pesticides than conventional farming. But does one thing necessarily lead to the other?

While the question of environmental impact is beyond the scope of this book, you can certainly apply the same principles about research presented in this chapter to other scientific questions, including this one. When you do, you'll likely find it hard to draw a clear-cut conclusion about whether one style of food production is better than the other. For example, one of the best summaries I've read on this issue reviewed a lot of the research and data and argued pretty convincingly that conventional farms are better at reducing erosion and tend to produce more food than organic farms. Organic farms, by contrast, tend to use less fertilizer and herbicides, have more fertile soil, use less energy, and lock more carbon away deep in the soil (which is important if you care about global warming). They're also more profitable for farmers. If the well-being of our environment is anywhere near as important to you as your own health, I encourage you to look into this research and judge for yourself.

Whether you're more interested in environmental or human health, it's important to remember that just because food is grown organically does not mean it's completely free of pesticides. In the United States, for instance, the government's standards do allow for pesticide use in the production of organic crops. Those regulations govern only the kinds of pesticides that are used, not how much. And what limited data we have suggest that, at least sometimes, farmers use organic pesticides much more liberally than conventional ones.

Organic pesticides are usually defined by how they were developed, not by how safe they are. One of the most well-known is rotenone, which can be used to kill insects and other pests. It's found naturally in some seeds, stems, and roots of plants, where it acts to inhibit infestations of pests such as leaf-eating caterpillars. Let me be clear: rotenone "inhibits" infestations by killing these creatures. And not just them; it's effective against all kinds of creatures, from beetles and spiders to worms, fish, and even mammals (although it's typically not used against them because it would require pretty large doses, which then might be dangerous to us). Its effectiveness makes it popular—that and the facts that it breaks down pretty quickly in the sun and it takes a lot to kill a human. But, just as with many other pesticides, some rat studies have shown that large enough doses of rotenone can be dangerous to mammals (in this case, by causing Parkinson's disease in rats), and the Food and Drug Administration has set limits on the amount of rotenone that is considered safe to consume. This is important because you can likely find trace amounts of rotenone, as well as other organic pesticides, in many organic foods.

I'm not telling you this to make you panic about rotenone or any other organic pesticide. You're no more likely to be harmed by being exposed to rotenone in organic foods than by being exposed to synthetic pesticides in conventionally grown foods. Rather, I'm telling you about rotenone because you should try to be consistent when weighing the pros and cons of all your choices, whether it's in regard to food or anything else. If you think that conventional pesticides are dangerous because they've been shown in animal studies to be harmful at high doses (as indeed they have been) and you don't trust the safe levels the U.S. government has set for these chemicals, you should feel the same concern about organic pesticides. Ditto for the environmental credits and debits. If your goal is to improve the environment and reduce damage caused by farming, presumably you want to use all the tools available to you — conventional or organic. Unfortunately, we seem to live in a world where it's one or the other.

I tend to be pretty relaxed about both types of foods, given the available evidence about them. But if you don't share that attitude, and you really want to eat foods that are grown using less fertilizer and herbicides, then GMOs — which can be engineered to require less of these substances — could be the answer. Of course, those are off-limits to many organic farmers, too.

Even though the "certified organic" designation has some positive benefits, I find the label itself less than helpful. For instance, one benefit of certified organic livestock, which I will happily acknowledge, is that the feed for animals raised organically doesn't include antibiotics. This means that fewer strains of drug-resistant bacteria will wind up in the meat we get from these animals. (The widespread use of antibiotics in the raising of animals has clearly contributed to the development of drug-resistant bacteria. "Widespread" may actually be an understatement. The FDA estimates that more kilograms of antibiotics are sold in the United States for food-producing animals than for people.)

If farmers want to be more cognizant of the antibiotics they use while raising animals, I'm all for it. But they don't need to raise certified organic livestock in order to do it.

THE BOTTOM LINE

The vast majority of food that's produced, sold, and consumed around the world is not organic. In the United States, only about 4% of all food that's sold is organic; the other 96% isn't. In many countries in Europe, that number is about twice as high, but still a minority of sales.

To some people, the ubiquity of conventionally grown foods is a tragedy — a catastrophe for the environment and for our health. The first of these concerns may be partially true, but the other is not. Organic foods are not essential to human health.

If there's a health benefit of organic foods, it's that they tend to help people eat better in general by encouraging them to eat more fruits and vegetables and steer clear of processed foods. My eating habits changed when we had the farm share. I started eating a wider variety of whole, fresh foods, which tasted amazing. That had little to do with how they were grown, or with their purported lack of chemicals, and everything to do with the fact that they were fresh and nonindustrial.

Once you've tasted a homegrown tomato from your garden or a local farm, the ones you purchase in the supermarket lose much of their appeal. Those tomatoes are designed primarily to stay fresh longer and be pretty much indestructible. The tomatoes you grow yourself are designed to taste awesome, even if they may be ugly. When food tastes better, we're more likely to eat it. *That's* an argument for organic foods that makes sense. I'm all for anything that helps us get people worldwide to eat more healthy foods and less crappy ones.

I'd never argue that organic foods are the only way to eat more healthily, especially given their expense. But many organic true believers don't share my scruples. Too often, they claim that organic foods are more nutritious and less dangerous than conventionally grown foods. Making such claims is counterproductive, and they're just not true.

Telling anyone who's eating conventionally grown fruits and vegetables that they're doing something wrong is not just terribly misguided; it's also potentially harmful. I'm thrilled that people who eat conventionally grown produce are eating fruits and vegetables at all. If you want to pay more for organic, my attitude is that it's a free country, and people can spend their money any way they like. But when it comes to telling others what to do, I'd like to see us spend more of our time and resources on getting the vast majority of people who aren't eating well to make better choices than to focus on getting people who are already eating pretty well to make a relatively meaningless change. At the end of the day, organic foods are a luxury—one that is simply not an option for most people.

Remember Norman Borlaug, the Nobel Prize–winning scientist I introduced back in chapter 6? Toward the end of his career, he argued that it was impossible to feed the world's growing population without modern chemical fertilizers and technology, and that without any evidence that avoiding these things provided a benefit, doing so would only reduce the chances that others might eat cheaply and easily, too. He called organic foods "ridiculous." I don't think you need to share that assessment in order to see his underlying point: for many people, conventionally grown foods are a godsend, not a curse.

CONCLUSION:
SIMPLE RULES FOR HEALTHY EATING

As I was writing this book, I'd often talk about it with family and friends. They'd ask me what the take-home message was. Sometimes I'd reply that I hoped the book would make people understand that the foods they're most concerned about aren't that dangerous. Other times I'd say that I hoped it would make people understand the difference between a small, relative risk to their health and a large, absolute risk — which is what people should really be worried about.

I'd also answer that I wanted readers to learn that we can't just look at one side of the equation when it comes to dietary health. We can't just talk about the potential harms of something. We also need to consider the potential benefits, because often the benefits — and quality of life is one of them — outweigh the very minimal harms, even if those harms do exist. Perhaps more than anything else, I found myself saying that I wanted readers to realize that we can't believe everything we hear about dietary health, even when it comes from scientists. The truth is much more complicated than any one study can reveal.

In time I have come to realize that these desires are all subsets of a bigger, even more important goal: to encourage people to develop a philosophy of eating that will help them be healthy both physically and mentally. When it comes to the foods we put in our bodies, the problem is overdoing it with specific foods, not enjoying any one food occasionally. We should allow ourselves to enjoy what we eat, and not be so concerned about it all the time.

Don't worry so much. That's the main message I want you to take away from this book.

Of course, it's much easier to tell people what *not* to do than what they should do. But books about food and nutrition inevitably need to provide some positive prescriptions — some "dos" as well as some "don'ts."

The truth is, prescriptions that are positive and also accurate are hard to make. As I've explained many times throughout this book, nutrition recommendations are seldom supported by science. I have taken many "experts" to task for telling people what to eat without having any research to back up their claims — or, worse, for telling people what to eat when the research starkly contradicts their advice. I am exceedingly wary of falling into the same trap.

So here's what I'm going to do: I'm going to give you the general rules that I live by. They're the ones I share with patients, friends, and family. They're the ones I endorse as a pediatrician and a health services researcher. But I acknowledge up front that they may apply only to healthy people without metabolic disorders (me, for instance — at least as far as I know).

These recommendations make sense to me, and they've helped me immensely, but they are not supported by the scientific weight of rigorous randomized controlled trials. Little in nutrition is. What good science there is, I've covered throughout this book. These rules are not "laws" and should not be treated as such. No specific nutrients are demonized, and none are held up as magic bullets.

Full disclosure: I did not invent most of these rules. I've developed them from reading the work of other experts and authorities, including what may be the most impressive national nutritional guidelines I've ever seen—Brazil's.* In addition, I've read almost all the comments from readers of my columns and viewers of my videos, and lots of them have good ideas, too. I've tried to bring together the best of all of this advice here.

Throughout this book, and in these rules, I've avoided treating any food like the devil. Many nutrition experts do this, and they may turn out to be right, but at this point I think the jury is still out.† I've therefore tried not to tell you to avoid anything completely. My experience has shown me that total abstinence rarely works, although anecdotes exist to support that practice. I think you'll find that lots of "diets" will work under the rules I've laid out here. They are much more flexible and, I hope, reasonable than what some might prescribe. They also aim to make you more conscious of what you're eating. It's far too easy these days to consume more than we intend to eat or really need, especially when we're eating out.

AARON'S RULES FOR
HEALTHY EATING

1. **Get as much of your nutrition as possible from a variety of completely unprocessed foods.** I've become convinced that one of the biggest problems we face when it comes to food has to do with processing. Pro-

---

* Seriously, you should check them out. They're amazing: http://bit.ly/1uB20iH.

† I've been struck by many recent books that identify carbohydrates, especially sugar, as the key nutrient of concern. But I'm not yet convinced scientists have proved that's the case. Until I am, I'm not going to tell you that low-carb is the way to go for everyone.

cessing has made it far too easy to cram stuff into our bodies. It's so much easier to drink that glass of juice than to eat an apple. It's easier to get carbs from bread or pasta than from flour. Packaged foods have been manipulated to be easy and fast, and from a health perspective, that is exactly what's wrong with them.

When you're buying foods at the market, focus on things that have not been cooked, prepared, or changed in any way: whole fruits and vegetables, eggs, and unadulterated beef, fish, and poultry. As much as possible, buy individual ingredients. If you have to look at a label on the side of a box to see what's in something you're considering buying, it's likely been processed.

This rule applies even to foods you may not think of as being heavily processed. For instance, brown rice is a less processed version of white rice. In general, you should choose whole grains such as brown rice over refined grains such as white rice. Similarly, you're far better off eating two apples than drinking the same 27 grams of sugar in an 8-ounce glass of apple juice. In fact, juice, in general, is a way to get all the calories without the fiber. Plus, the work of eating the whole ingredient might slow you down a bit and make you less likely to overconsume. When it comes to food, "quick and easy" is not necessarily a selling point.

2. **Eat lightly processed foods less often.** You're not going to make everything yourself. It's very unlikely, for instance, that you're always going to make your own pasta. You're not going to grind your own flour or extract your own oil. That's fine. These foods are really okay, but they're meant to be eaten along with unpro-

cessed foods. You can have them, but try to eat less of them than you do of completely unprocessed foods.

3. **Eat heavily processed foods even less often.** There's little high-quality evidence that even the most processed foods are dangerous when eaten in modest quantities. In keeping with the theme of this book, I wouldn't recommend that you banish them completely from your diet. Hot bread with butter is close to heaven. The key is to keep your consumption of heavily processed foods to a minimum, because, again, they make consuming too easy. Heavily processed foods include most breads, chips, cookies, and cereals. Even when you make these things at home, the ingredients they come from are often heavily processed, and the act of combining them adds another layer of processing. And, of course, lots of processed foods, such as candy and fast food, are not going to be made at home, and should also be eaten less often. As I've noted in previous chapters, heavily processed meat is the food most associated with the worst health outcomes, but that evidence should be taken with a grain of salt (literally, if you like). You can have all these things; just try to have less of them than other types of foods.

4. **Eat as much home-cooked food as possible, preparing it according to rules 1, 2, and 3.** Eating at home allows you to avoid processed ingredients more easily. It allows you full control over what you eat, and it allows you to choose the flavors you prefer. You're also much less likely to stuff yourself silly if you eat home-cooked food.

This is the recommendation that gets me into the most trouble with other food experts. They claim that this is the advice of an "elitist," that cooking at home is much harder than I think, and that many people just can't do it. They'll even throw research at me that says so. I acknowledge that this is true. Cooking well, and cooking healthily, takes effort. Behavioral change takes repetition and practice. Both also, unfortunately, take time. It even takes money, and I support policies that seek to overcome all these barriers.

But practically everyone can prepare tasty, healthy food if they commit themselves to doing it. I'm sometimes struck by how many of the people who complain that they don't have time to cook seem to have hours to devote to exercise. The amount of time they spend getting to where they work out, exercising, showering and dressing again, and then getting back home or to work, dwarfs the time and effort they are willing to put into preparing what they eat. Exercise is not the key to maintaining a healthy weight. What you eat is so much more important. If these people would just dedicate some of the time they spend working out to working in the kitchen, I bet they'd see much more impressive results. (Don't get me wrong: exercise is important for many reasons besides regulating body weight. You should be physically active. But you should also maintain a healthy diet.)

5. **Use salt and fats, including butter and oil, as needed in food preparation.** Things like salt and fat aren't the enemy. They are often necessary in the preparation of tasty, satisfying food. When I was a kid, I thought Brussels sprouts were just terrible. But it turns out that if you

broil them with some oil and sea salt, they are unbelievably good. If my parents had prepared them that way, I
would have eaten a lot more of them, rather than filling
myself up with other, less healthy foods.

I can't say this enough: seasoning is often what makes
healthy foods taste good. I'm mystified by how people
will make main dishes calling for twenty ingredients and
requiring ten different steps, but then leave the vegetables they serve on the side plain and dry. Don't do that.
Even if it takes some supposedly "bad" ingredients to
make the healthy ones more palatable, use them. The
scolds who want you to avoid butter, salt, or MSG, or to
eat your salad with no dressing, don't get that this often makes food unpalatable. Seasonings are almost always the key ingredients in everything delicious. Don't
be afraid of them, but don't go crazy with them either.
The key here is moderation. Use what you need but no
more.

6. **When you do eat out, try to eat at restaurants that
   follow the same rules.** You're not going to cook every
   night. We don't in our house. Every Friday we go out to
   dinner as a family, and every Saturday my wife and I go
   out for an adult dinner.* Even when we dine out, however, we try to eat at restaurants that create most of
   their menu items from unprocessed foods.

   Many restaurants today follow rules 1, 2, 3, and 5 —
   but not all restaurants do. You'll often be served breads,
   sauces, soups, and pasta that have been heavily pro-

---

* I'm serious about this. Our Saturday night adult dinner is pretty much a holiday in the Carroll household. I think it's the key to a happy marriage, and when I someday write my book on
healthy relationships, this will be an essential factor.

cessed. So be mindful of what you're ordering, and follow rules 1–3 even when eating out. You know what's in a baked potato. You have no idea what's in the sauce-covered potato soufflé. Some processing is fine, but try to keep it to a minimum.

7. **Drink mostly water, but some alcohol, coffee, and other beverages are fine.** There's simply no doubt that water is the liquid that we were meant to consume. It's the beverage of choice for pretty much every other mammal on the planet. That doesn't mean you can't enjoy other drinks once in a while, too. As I've pointed out repeatedly in this book, you can find a study to show that *anything* either prevents or causes cancer—alcohol and coffee included. The preponderance of evidence supports the consumption of a moderate amount of most beverages that aren't purely water. Even without taking quality of life into account, you can easily make an argument (as I have in this book) that the benefits of occasionally enjoying many of these drinks outweigh the harms.

8. **Treat all calorie-containing beverages as you would alcohol.** The counterpoint to rule 7 is that you can't ignore what's in the beverages you're drinking. This rule applies to every drink with calories, including milk. Liquid nutrition is so easy to consume that we often end up consuming too much of it. Caloric beverages are fine in moderation, but keep them to a minimum. You can have them because you like them, but you shouldn't drink them as if you *need* them.

9. **Eat with other people, especially people you care about, as often as possible.** If you remember only one

rule on this list, I hope it's this one. Every time I see or hear something that's trying to make us afraid of food, make eating somehow miserable, or push an unpleasant diet that's supposedly "good for you," it makes me angry. Recommendations like these make it more difficult to enjoy food with other people, and that's a travesty. Eating together has been one of the rituals that, since time immemorial, defines groups that care about one another. Eating together is how we celebrate. It's how we mourn. It's how we fall in love. How can we tell anyone to deny themselves this elemental pleasure?

I almost always eat lunch by myself at my desk. It's sad. I don't like it. I leave the office every day at five p.m. on the nose, however, because I eat dinner every night with my family. That's the highlight of my day. When I have to travel, I'm almost never gone over a weekend, because missing dinner out with my family or my wife and friends is pretty much unthinkable.

Aimee and I aren't particularly spend-happy people, but that rule completely vanishes when it comes to food. When we travel, especially with friends, the most important thing we plan is where we are going to eat. I've been to many of the best restaurants in the United States, but I also love the little holes-in-the-wall that only the locals know. One way or another, I love to try new food — but always with people I care about. Without hesitation, I can rattle off my top five meals of all time, what was going on in my life at the time, and with whom I was eating. Companionship is the cornerstone of a healthy diet.

Eating with other people has benefits beyond nutrition. It will make you more likely to cook. It will probably make you eat more slowly. It will also make you happy. Do it.

THE BOTTOM LINE

There are no pictures in our house of Aimee and me before our kids were born. The reason is that neither of us is particularly proud of our weight, or our overall health, back then. She jokes that the pictures of herself right before Jacob was born are of "the woman who ate Aimee." The pictures of me are harder to joke about. I wasn't taking good care of myself.

Both of us are much thinner and healthier now. People often ask what we did to lose weight. The truth is that there was no magic bullet. Rather, simply following the rules I've outlined here has proven to be effective and sustainable for us.

I've tried a variety of diets in my time. Some were "low-fat." Some involved calorie counting. Most recently, I've been experimenting with a low-carb meal plan. But I find that the most dramatically effective diet I've ever followed was more subtle than any of these. It was when our family expanded from two people to three, then four, then five. As it did, Aimee started cooking more, and, not coincidentally, we increased our vegetable intake, lowered our consumption of pasta and bread, and became more aware of the calories we were consuming in beverages as well as solid foods.

Years ago, I was sitting in synagogue during a holiday, and our rabbi gave a sermon on the rules of being kosher. They're complicated, and they were written at a time when people's eating habits were very different than they are today. Food safety was a significant issue back then. For example, dairy products could spoil easily and needed to be kept away from meat. But my rabbi didn't focus on the importance of following this rule or that rule, but on the way those dietary rules encourage us to be conscious of what we are consuming. We are, after all, what we eat.

This does not mean that we should judge what others eat. One of my closest friends avoids carbohydrates like the plague and has seen remarkable results. Another was a pescatarian — eating no meat except fish — for a year and was very happy with that. I, by contrast, avoid no food groups in particular. In fact, I vary my diet quite considerably from year to year.

In general, I've found that it's impossible to tell anyone how much he or she should eat. People have different requirements, and it's important for us to listen to our bodies so that we know when we should eat and when we should stop.

People also have various dietary issues. Some may have real problems consuming even the smallest amount of a certain nutrient. Others may be intolerant of particular foods because of allergies or sensitivities. It will most likely take a bit of experimentation, on an individual level, to find the actual diet that works for you. But the rules I've provided should allow for a wide variety of foods that you can eat enjoyably. At least, I hope so.

As with all rules, mine are sometimes meant to be broken. When my family goes on vacation, I eat whatever I want. When I'm in a fancy restaurant, I eat what the chef recommends. On Thanksgiving, all bets are off. (I love pie.) Give yourself a pass on special occasions like these. It's the rest of the year that matters, not the few times you let yourself go.

I would be remiss if I didn't note that you should, of course, talk to your own physician before making any big changes in how you eat. You need to know your own medical risks to figure out what's best for you. But when you're talking to your physician — and when you're thinking about food in general — I hope you'll think critically, ask questions, and demand the evidence for what you are told.

Eating is one of the great joys of life. Don't let people use misinformation or bad science to deprive you of the pleasure of good food. If they tell you that you need to drastically change your eating habits, or that you need to avoid this or that food completely, be skeptical; that's almost never the case. You can eat things you love and still live a long and healthy life. Let this book be your guide.

ACKNOWLEDGMENTS

First, I want to thank my employer for the past fourteen years, Indiana University School of Medicine. If you had told me before I came to Indiana that I would live in the Midwest, I would have laughed. If you had told me that I'd be here for more than a decade, I might have cried. But Indiana has become my home, and that is in no small part because I have the best job in the world. Besides allowing me to do the research and teaching that I love, my many bosses have provided me the space to pursue additional activities (like writing) that would normally require a leave of absence or a vacation. I'm grateful for their continued support and for their faith in my work.

Two work-related people deserve special mention: Kat Coppedge, my assistant of many years and one of the few people who never fears to tell me the truth, and Jen Buddenbaum, my right hand for more than a decade and the most indispensable employee anyone could ever have.

I want to thank all of my *Upshot* colleagues at the *New York Times*. My editors, Damon Darlin, Laura Chang, Kevin Quealy, Amanda Cox, and David Leonhardt, helped to make many of the columns that formed the basis for this book stronger and more enjoyable. Margot Sanger-Katz also provided helpful feedback and ideas for many of those columns as well.

I would never have had the opportunity to do any of that writing if not for the blog *The Incidental Economist*. When I started writing about health policy and research there, I think our traffic was likely counted in the tens. Seeing it today is simply unbelievable. None of that would have been possible without Austin Frakt, my constant companion on this crazy writing journey. I also need to thank Adrianna McIntyre and Nicholas Bagley, both of whom were kind enough to read the proposal for this book and to help make the blog one of the most widely read health policy destinations in the world.

In 2009, I was a guest on *Stand Up! with Pete Dominick,* on SiriusXM, which soon became a weekly occurrence. Years later, Pete is now one of my best friends and biggest supporters. He's the one who encouraged me to start a blog in the first place, and he's part of the gang that believes I'm always capable of more. I'm eternally grateful.

Another opportunity that changed my world was the YouTube show *Healthcare Triage.* Many of the chapters in this book came out of episodes of that show, and working on it has been one of the great joys of my life. I am forever indebted to Stan Muller and Mark Olsen, both of whose contributions to my work are innumerable.

That show only came into being because of John Green, whose support and friendship are truly *the* reason this book happened. He and his wife, Sarah Urist Green, have become great friends of ours, and I will forever be thankful for the random Twitter user who connected us after John did a video on why health care costs so much in the United States (using lots of research I'd done for my blog). I thought I was done with books, but John's constant prodding and pushing made this thing happen. He introduced me to Jodi Reamer, my agent, another person without whom none of this would have been possible. Her genuine and thoughtful advice shaped this book from start to finish, and the final product is due in no small part to her skill and wit.

On that note, I also need to acknowledge my editor, Alex Littlefield, and his editorial associate, Pilar Garcia-Brown, without whose help this book would have been nowhere near as good as it is. I've learned over the course of my career that great editing makes for great writing, and they deserve a lot of credit for what you've just read.

Providing reassurance and constant faith in my talents are friends who may as well be family. Todd and Linda Mauer, and their children, Alexis, Tessa, and Bella, were our first true friends in Indianapolis, and they have held that position for many years. More recent additions, but no less loved, are Jim and Ali Fleischer, and their kids, Ethan, Spencer, and Madi. They make our annual trips to Michigan something I look forward to instead of tolerating. David and Jackie Barrett and Greg and Megan Maurer have also been companions on some of our best eating ventures, and I can forever count on them to teach me something about food or wine. I can also count on David and Greg to tolerate my eye rolls, Todd to rile me up about some fake bit of science, and Jim to laugh at my jokes. Friends who know how to push your buttons and make you feel talented are indispensable.

Another coterie that deserves specific mention is my gaming group: Tyson, Kurt, Tim, Adam, Chad, Ben, and Hayden — as well as Stan Muller and my two boys. Seeing them is one of the highlights of my week. Plus, no one is better at spotting crappy research and bringing it to my attention than this gang.

My parents, Stan and Shelley Carroll, have always believed that there's nothing I cannot do, even when I might have doubted myself. My in-laws, Michael and Sharon Schuman, have taken up that mantle as well. The love and support of my siblings and siblings-in-law has been indispensable as well.

A special thank-you goes to my brother, David, though. He's the only person I talk to on the phone almost every day. His support is priceless. In 1994, we drove 8,500 miles together in a car over the summer. He's the only person in the world I could do that with.

Last, but certainly not least, I need to talk about my family. I always knew I would love my kids, but I never expected that I'd have three smaller people living in my house that I would like so much, too. It can't be easy to live with me all the time, but they do so with grace. They tolerate my faults and lift me up when I'm down. Most impressively, they never say no to a game, especially old-school *Mario Party*. When I bought that game almost two decades ago, I never imagined I'd someday have built-in companions who would play at the drop of a hat. Jacob is a better man than I am. Noah is the man I wish I could be. Sydney just rocks my world. May she never stop wanting to hold my hand. I love them (and even Sydney's hamster, Gizmo Fluffybottom) so very much.

And then there's Aimee. It's hard to know where to start. Words fail to convey how much I owe her. The only reason I've been able to do the things I've done is because she's there to keep everything else going. She's the most organized, most proficient, and most caring person I know. She's the reason my kids are so great. She's the reason I look presentable. She's the reason I have friends, a social life, and new experiences. I love her more than I can say, and if I've done anything you like in · the past twenty years, you can thank her for it. It's all because of her.

I hope she knows that.

NOTES

INTRODUCTION

page

xviii *my first official publication:* A. E. Carroll, M. M. Garrison, and D. A. Christakis, "A Systematic Review of Nonpharmacological and Nonsurgical Therapies for Gastroesophageal Reflux in Infants," *Archives of Pediatrics & Adolescent Medicine* 156, no. 2 (2002): 109–13.

xxvi *study published in the* Journal of Nutrition: S. K. Raatz, L. K. Johnson, and M. J. Picklo, "Consumption of Honey, Sucrose, and High-Fructose Corn Syrup Produces Similar Metabolic Effects in Glucose-Tolerant and -Intolerant Individuals," *Journal of Nutrition* 145, no. 10 (2015): 2265–72.

xxvii *This fact is vividly demonstrated:* N. Wiebe, R. Padwal, C. Field, S. Marks, R. Jacobs, and M. Tonelli, "A Systematic Review on the Effect of Sweeteners on Glycemic Response and Clinically Relevant Outcomes," *BMC Medicine* 9 (2011): 123.

xxviii *study published in the journal* Frontiers in Nutrition: V. L. Choo and J. L. Sievenpiper, "The Ecologic Validity of Fructose Feeding Trials: Supraphysiological Feeding of Fructose in Human Trials Requires Careful Consideration When Drawing Conclusions on Cardiometabolic Risk," *Frontiers in Nutrition* 2 (2015): 12.

xxix *come from prisons or mental hospitals:* O. Turpeinen, M. Pekkarinen, M. Miettinen, R. Elosuo, and E. Paavilainen, "Dietary Prevention of Coronary Heart Disease: The Finnish Mental Hospital Study," *International Journal of Epidemiology* 8, no. 2 (1979): 99–118.

xxxii *millions of papers get published:* Mark Ware, *The STM Report: An Overview of Scientific and Scholarly Journal Publishing,* 4th ed. (The Hague: International Association of Scientific, Technical and Medical Publishers, 2015), 6, http://www.stm-assoc.org/2015_02_20_STM_Report_2015.pdf.

If you're inclined to hate meat: M. Song, T. T. Fung, F. B. Hu, W. C. Willett, V. D. Longo, A. T. Chan, et al., "Association of Animal and Plant Protein Intake with All-Cause and Cause-Specific Mortality," *JAMA Internal Medicine* 176, no. 10 (2016): 1453–63.

If you're inclined to love meat: K.S.D. Kothapalli, K. Ye, M. S. Gadgil, S. E. Carlson, K. O. O'Brien, J. Y. Zhang, et al., "Positive Selection on a Regulatory Insertion-Deletion Polymorphism in FADS2 Influences Apparent Endogenous Synthesis of Arachidonic Acid," *Molecular Biology and Evolution* 33, no. 7 (2016): 1726–39.

research investigating fifty common ingredients: J. D. Schoenfeld and J. P. Ioannidis, "Is

Everything We Eat Associated with Cancer? A Systematic Cookbook Review," *American Journal of Clinical Nutrition* 97, no. 1 (2013): 127–34.

1. BUTTER

3   *sound the death knell for trans fats:* D. Mozaffarian, M. B. Katan, A. Ascherio, M. J. Stampfer, and W. C. Willett, "Trans Fatty Acids and Cardiovascular Disease," *New England Journal of Medicine* 354, no. 15 (2006): 1601–13.

companies had to start explicitly labeling: Food and Drug Administration, "Food Labeling: Trans Fatty Acids in Nutrition Labeling, Nutrient Content Claims, and Health Claims," 68 Fed. Reg. 41433–41506 (July 11, 2003), https://www.fda.gov/ohrms/dockets/98fr/03-17525.htm.

4   *the tiny amounts that remain:* M. E. Levine, J. A. Suarez, S. Brandhorst, P. Balasubramanian, C. W. Cheng, F. Madia, et al., "Low Protein Intake Is Associated with a Major Reduction in IGF-1, Cancer, and Overall Mortality in the 65 and Younger but Not Older Population," *Cell Metabolism* 19, no. 3 (2014): 407–17.

could prevent about 20,000 heart attacks: J. T. Cohen, D. C. Bellinger, and B. A. Shaywitz, "A Quantitative Analysis of Prenatal Methyl Mercury Exposure and Cognitive Development," *American Journal of Preventive Medicine* 29, no. 4 (2005): 353–65.

FDA issued a Federal Register *notice:* E. Oken, R. O. Wright, K. P. Kleinman, D. Bellinger, C. J. Amarasiriwardena, H. Hu, et al., "Maternal Fish Consumption, Hair Mercury, and Infant Cognition in a U.S. Cohort," *Environmental Health Perspectives* 113, no. 10 (2005): 1376–80.

Minnesota Coronary Experiment: C. E. Ramsden, D. Zamora, S. Majchrzak-Hong, K. R. Faurot, S. K. Broste, R. P. Frantz, et al., "Re-evaluation of the Traditional Diet-Heart Hypothesis: Analysis of Recovered Data from Minnesota Coronary Experiment (1968–73)," *BMJ* 353 (2016): i1246.

6   *an analysis of recovered data:* C. E. Ramsden, D. Zamora, B. Leelarthaepin, S. F. Majchrzak-Hong, K. R. Faurot, C. M. Suchindran, et al., "Use of Dietary Linoleic Acid for Secondary Prevention of Coronary Heart Disease and Death: Evaluation of Recovered Data from the Sydney Diet Heart Study and Updated Meta-analysis," *BMJ* 346 (2013): e8707.

researchers conducted a meta-analysis: Ramsden et al., "Re-evaluation of the Traditional Diet-Heart Hypothesis."

reduce people's rates of coronary heart disease: D. Mozaffarian, R. Micha, and S. Wallace, "Effects on Coronary Heart Disease of Increasing Polyunsaturated Fat in Place of Saturated Fat: A Systematic Review and Meta-analysis of Randomized Controlled Trials," *PLOS Medicine* 7, no. 3 (2010): e1000252.

a 2015 systematic review: L. Hooper, N. Martin, A. Abdelhamid, and G. Davey Smith, "Reduction in Saturated Fat Intake for Cardiovascular Disease," *Cochrane Database of Systematic Reviews*, no. 6 (2015).

a 2014 study published in the Annals of Internal Medicine: R. Chowdhury, S. Warnakula, S. Kunutsor, F. Crowe, H. A. Ward, L. Johnson, et al., "Association of Dietary, Circulating, and Supplement Fatty Acids with Coronary Risk: A Systematic Review and Meta-analysis," *Annals of Internal Medicine* 160, no. 6 (2014): 398–406.

7   *the most influential scientist:* "Ancel Keys," The Seven Countries Study, 2016, http://
     www.sevencountriesstudy.com/about-the-study/investigators/ancel-keys/.
8   *a phenomenon called* publication bias: F. Song, L. Hooper, and Y. K. Loke, "Publication
     Bias: What Is It? How Do We Measure It? How Do We Avoid It?," *Open Access Journal
     of Clinical Trials* 5 (2013): 71–81.
     less likely to be published: F. Song, S. Parekh, L. Hooper, Y. K. Loke, and J. Ryder, "Dis-
     semination and Publication of Research Findings: An Updated Review of Related Bi-
     ases," *Health Technology Assessment* 14, no. 8 (2010): 234.
     researchers simply don't write up their work: A. E. Carroll, C. M. Sox, B. A. Tarini, S. Rin-
     gold, and D. A. Christakis, "Does Presentation Format at the Pediatric Academic Socie-
     ties' Annual Meeting Predict Subsequent Publication?," *Pediatrics* 112, no. 6 (2003): 1238.
9   *low-fat diets do not outperform:* D. K. Tobias, M. Chen, J. E. Manson, D. S. Ludwig, W.
     Willett, and F. B. Hu, "Effect of Low-Fat Diet Interventions Versus Other Diet Interven-
     tions on Long-Term Weight Change in Adults: A Systematic Review and Meta-analy-
     sis," *Lancet Diabetes & Endocrinology* 3, no. 12 (2015):968–79.
     well-designed two-year study: I. Shai, D. Schwarzfuchs, Y. Henkin, D. R. Shahar, S. Wit-
     kow, I. Greenberg, et al., "Weight Loss with a Low-Carbohydrate, Mediterranean, or
     Low-Fat Diet," *New England Journal of Medicine* 359, no. 3 (2008): 229–41.
10   *American Academy of Pediatrics:* A. I. Eidelman, R. J. Schanler, M. Johnston, S. Landers,
     L. Noble, K. Szucs, et al., "Breastfeeding and the Use of Human Milk," *Pediatrics* 129, no.
     3 (2012): e827–41.
     Institute of Medicine: Institute of Medicine, Committee on Obesity Prevention Policies
     for Young Children, *Early Childhood Obesity Prevention Policies,* ed. L. L. Birch, A. C.
     Burns, and L. Parker (Washington, DC: National Academies Press, 2011), xii.
     World Health Organization: "Exclusive Breastfeeding," World Health Organization,
     http://www.who.int/nutrition/topics/exclusive_breastfeeding/en/.
     3 cups a day: "All About the Dairy Group," ChooseMyPlate.gov, https://www.choosemy
     plate.gov/dairy.
     Proponents of the Paleo Diet: Loren Cordain, "Dairy: Milking It for All It's Worth," The
     Paleo Diet, http://thepaleodiet.com/dairy-milking-worth/.
     no adults or older children consumed milk: A. Curry, "Archaeology: The Milk Revolu-
     tion," *Nature* 500, no. 7460 (2013): 20–22.
11   *published a meta-analysis:* H. A. Bischoff-Ferrari, B. Dawson-Hughes, J. A. Baron, J. A.
     Kanis, E. J. Orav, H. B. Staehelin, et al., "Milk Intake and Risk of Hip Fracture in Men
     and Women: A Meta-analysis of Prospective Cohort Studies," *Journal of Bone and Min-
     eral Research* 26, no. 4 (2011): 833–39.
     It wasn't: D. Feskanich, H. A. Bischoff-Ferrari, A. Frazier, and W. C. Willett, "Milk Con-
     sumption During Teenage Years and Risk of Hip Fractures in Older Adults," *JAMA Pe-
     diatrics* 168, no. 1 (2014): 54–60.
     increased risk of fractures: K. Michaëlsson, A. Wolk, S. Langenskiöld, S. Basu, E. Wa-
     rensjö Lemming, H. Melhus, et al., "Milk Intake and Risk of Mortality and Fractures in
     Women and Men: Cohort Studies," *BMJ* 349 (2014): g6015.
     A 2007 meta-analysis: H. A. Bischoff-Ferrari, B. Dawson-Hughes, J. A. Baron, P. Burck-
     hardt, R. Li, D. Spiegelman, et al., "Calcium Intake and Hip Fracture Risk in Men and
     Women: A Meta-analysis of Prospective Cohort Studies and Randomized Controlled
     Trials," *American Journal of Clinical Nutrition* 86, no. 6 (2007): 1780–90.

12   *the effects of vitamin D supplementation:* I. R. Reid, M. J. Bolland, and A. Grey, "Effects of Vitamin D Supplements on Bone Mineral Density: A Systematic Review and Meta-analysis," *Lancet* 383, no. 9912 (2014): 146–55.

13   *increase dairy consumption:* Michael Moss, "While Warning About Fat, U.S. Pushes Cheese Sales," *New York Times,* November 6, 2010, http://www.nytimes.com/2010/11/07/us/07fat.html.

14   *a protective effect against diabetes:* D. Gao, N. Ning, C. Wang, Y. Wang, Q. Li, Z. Meng, et al., "Dairy Products Consumption and Risk of Type 2 Diabetes: Systematic Review and Dose-Response Meta-analysis," *PLOS ONE* 8, no. 9 (2013): e73965.

      a positive effect on cardiovascular health: P. C. Elwood, J. E. Pickering, D. I. Givens, and J. E. Gallacher, "The Consumption of Milk and Dairy Foods and the Incidence of Vascular Disease and Diabetes: An Overview of the Evidence," *Lipids* 45, no. 10 (2010): 925–39.

      not associated with significant weight gain: K. J. Murphy, G. E. Crichton, K. A. Dyer, A. M. Coates, T. L. Pettman, C. Milte, et al., "Dairy Foods and Dairy Protein Consumption Is Inversely Related to Markers of Adiposity in Obese Men and Women," *Nutrients* 5, no. 11 (2013): 4665–84.

      that's not true either: P. C. Elwood, D. I. Givens, A. D. Beswick, A. M. Fehily, J. E. Pickering, and J. Gallacher, "The Survival Advantage of Milk and Dairy Consumption: An Overview of Evidence from Cohort Studies of Vascular Diseases, Diabetes and Cancer," *Journal of the American College of Nutrition* 27, no. 6 (2008): 723s–34s.

15   *replacing saturated fats with polyunsaturated fats:* "Scientific Report of the 2015 Dietary Guidelines Advisory Committee," part D, chapter 6 (U.S. Department of Agriculture and U.S. Department of Health and Human Services, first print, February 2015), https://health.gov/dietaryguidelines/2015-scientific-report/11-chapter-6/.

2. MEAT

19   *first published in 1983:* M. Kushi with A. Jack, *The Cancer Prevention Diet: Michio Kushi's Nutritional Blueprint for the Prevention and Relief of Disease,* 1st ed. (New York: St. Martin's Press, 1983).

20   *eating more meat than they have:* U.S. Department of Agriculture, *Agriculture Fact Book* (Washington, DC: Government Printing Office, 2003), 15.

21   *"An optimal diet for preventing disease":* D. Ornish, "The Myth of High-Protein Diets," *New York Times,* March 23, 2015, https://www.nytimes.com/2015/03/23/opinion/the-myth-of-high-protein-diets.html.

22   *He mentioned one particular study:* M. E. Levine, J. A. Suarez, S. Brandhorst, P. Balasubramanian, C. W. Cheng, F. Madia, et al., "Low Protein Intake Is Associated with a Major Reduction in IGF-1, Cancer, and Overall Mortality in the 65 and Younger but Not Older Population," *Cell Metabolism* 19, no. 3 (2014): 407–17.

23   *according to USDA guidelines:* U.S. Department of Health and Human Services and U.S. Department of Agriculture, *2015–2020 Dietary Guidelines for Americans,* 8th ed. (December 2015), https://health.gov/dietaryguidelines/2015/guidelines/.

25   *a decrease of 0.7 point:* J. T. Cohen, D. C. Bellinger, and B. A. Shaywitz, "A Quantitative

Analysis of Prenatal Methyl Mercury Exposure and Cognitive Development," *American Journal of Preventive Medicine* 29, no. 4 (2005): 353–65.

associated with smarter kids: E. Oken, R. O. Wright, K. P. Kleinman, D. Bellinger, C. J. Amarasiriwardena, H. Hu, et al., "Maternal Fish Consumption, Hair Mercury, and Infant Cognition in a U.S. Cohort," *Environmental Health Perspectives* 113, no. 10 (2005): 1376–80.

26   *In 2006, two researchers:* D. Mozaffarian and E. B. Rimm, "Fish Intake, Contaminants, and Human Health: Evaluating the Risks and the Benefits," *JAMA* 296, no. 15 (2006): 1885–99.

27   *esophageal cancer:* G. Jiang, B. Li, X. Liao, and C. Zhong, "Poultry and Fish Intake and Risk of Esophageal Cancer: A Meta-analysis of Observational Studies," *Asia-Pacific Journal of Clinical Oncology* 12, no. 1 (2016): e82–91.

ovarian cancer: F. Kolahdooz, J. C. van der Pols, C. J. Bain, G. C. Marks, M. C. Hughes, D. C. Whiteman, et al., "Meat, Fish, and Ovarian Cancer Risk: Results from 2 Australian Case-Control Studies, a Systematic Review, and Meta-analysis," *American Journal of Clinical Nutrition* 91, no. 6 (2010): 1752–63.

colon cancer: B. Xu, J. Sun, Y. Sun, L. Huang, Y. Tang, and Y. Yuan, "No Evidence of Decreased Risk of Colorectal Adenomas with White Meat, Poultry, and Fish Intake: A Meta-analysis of Observational Studies," *Annals of Epidemiology* 23, no. 4 (2013): 215–22.

lower risk of developing diabetes: K. Esposito, C. M. Kastorini, D. B. Panagiotakos, and D. Giugliano, "Prevention of Type 2 Diabetes by Dietary Patterns: A Systematic Review of Prospective Studies and Meta-analysis," *Metabolic Syndrome and Related Disorders* 8, no. 6 (2010): 471–76.

including heart attacks and death: R. Estruch, E. Ros, J. Salas-Salvadó, M.-I. Covas, D. Corella, F. Arós, et al., "Primary Prevention of Cardiovascular Disease with a Mediterranean Diet," *New England Journal of Medicine* 368, no. 14 (2013): 1279–90.

nutritional components of poultry are favorable: F. Marangoni, G. Corsello, C. Cricelli, N. Ferrara, A. Ghiselli, L. Lucchin, et al., "Role of Poultry Meat in a Balanced Diet Aimed at Maintaining Health and Wellbeing: An Italian Consensus Document," *Food & Nutrition Research* 59 (2015): 27606.

not been associated with cancer: P. R. Carr, V. Walter, H. Brenner, and M. Hoffmeister, "Meat Subtypes and Their Association with Colorectal Cancer: Systematic Review and Meta-analysis," *International Journal of Cancer* 138, no. 2 (2016): 293–302.

associated with a decreased risk: Esposito et al., "Prevention of Type 2 Diabetes by Dietary Patterns."

28   *no harmful effects of eating poultry:* M. S. Farvid, A. F. Malekshah, A. Pourshams, H. Poustchi, S. G. Sepanlou, M. Sharafkhah, et al., "Dietary Protein Sources and All-Cause and Cause-Specific Mortality: The Golestan Cohort Study in Iran," *American Journal of Preventive Medicine* 52, no. 2 (2017): 237–48.

a meta-analysis of prospective: J. Wu, R. Zeng, J. Huang, X. Li, J. Zhang, J. C.-M. Ho, et al., "Dietary Protein Sources and Incidence of Breast Cancer: A Dose-Response Meta-analysis of Prospective Studies," *Nutrients* 8, no. 11 (2016): 730.

lower rates of the progression of the disease: K. M. Wilson, L. A. Mucci, B. F. Drake, M. A. Preston, M. J. Stampfer, E. Giovannucci, et al., "Meat, Fish, Poultry, and Egg Intake at

Diagnosis and Risk of Prostate Cancer Progression," *Cancer Prevention Research* 9, no. 12 (2016): 933–41.

National Institutes of Health–AARP Diet and Health Study: R. Sinha, A. J. Cross, B. I. Graubard, M. F. Leitzmann, and A. Schatzkin, "Meat Intake and Mortality: A Prospective Study of over Half a Million People," *Archives of Internal Medicine* 169, no. 6 (2009): 562–71.

29   *study published in 2012:* K. J. Murphy, R. L. Thomson, A. M. Coates, J. D. Buckley, and P.R.C. Howe, "Effects of Eating Fresh Lean Pork on Cardiometabolic Health Parameters," *Nutrients* 4, no. 7 (2012): 711–23.

did not observe any significant differences: K. J. Murphy, B. Parker, K. A. Dyer, C. R. Davis, A. Coates, J. D. Buckley, et al., "A Comparison of Regular Consumption of Fresh Lean Pork, Beef and Chicken on Body Composition: A Randomized Cross-Over Trial," *Nutrients* 6, no. 2 (2014): 682–96.

extra pork, extra iron, or a control diet: J. O. McArthur, N. M. Gough, P. Petocz, and S. Samman, "Inclusion of Pork Meat in the Diets of Young Women Reduces Their Intakes of Energy-Dense, Nutrient-Poor Foods: Results from a Randomized Controlled Trial," *Nutrients* 6, no. 6 (2014): 2320–32.

30   *beef, shrimp, or mixed sources of protein:* N. Stettler, M. M. Murphy, L. M. Barraj, K. M. Smith, and R. S. Ahima, "Systematic Review of Clinical Studies Related to Pork Intake and Metabolic Syndrome or Its Components," *Diabetes, Metabolic Syndrome and Obesity: Targets and Therapy* 6 (2013): 347–57.

results weren't that striking: A.M.J. Gilsing, M. P. Weijenberg, L.A.E. Hughes, T. Ambergen, P. C. Dagnelie, R. A. Goldbohm, et al., "Longitudinal Changes in BMI in Older Adults Are Associated with Meat Consumption Differentially, by Type of Meat Consumed," *Journal of Nutrition* 142, no. 2 (2012): 340–49.

a 2014 meta-analysis: S. C. Larsson and N. Orsini, "Red Meat and Processed Meat Consumption and All-Cause Mortality: A Meta-analysis," *American Journal of Epidemiology* 179, no. 3 (2014): 282–89.

32   *World Health Organization's 2015 Q&A:* "Q&A on the Carcinogenicity of the Consumption of Red Meat and Processed Meat," World Health Organization, October 2015, http://www.who.int/features/qa/cancer-red-meat/en/.

meta-analysis of cohort studies published in PLOS ONE: D.S.M. Chan, R. Lau, D. Aune, R. Vieira, D. C. Greenwood, E. Kampman, et al., "Red and Processed Meat and Colorectal Cancer Incidence: Meta-analysis of Prospective Studies," *PLOS ONE* 6, no. 6 (2011): e20456.

33   *The Polyp Prevention Trial:* E. Lanza, B. Yu, G. Murphy, P. S. Albert, B. Caan, J. R. Marshall, et al., "The Polyp Prevention Trial Continued Follow-Up Study: No Effect of a Low-Fat, High-Fiber, High-Fruit, and -Vegetable Diet on Adenoma Recurrence Eight Years After Randomization," *Cancer Epidemiology, Biomarkers & Prevention* 16, no. 9 (2007): 1745–52.

The Women's Health Initiative: S. A. Beresford, K. C. Johnson, C. Ritenbaugh, N. L. Lasser, L. G. Snetselaar, H. R. Black, et al., "Low-Fat Dietary Pattern and Risk of Colorectal Cancer: The Women's Health Initiative Randomized Controlled Dietary Modification Trial," *JAMA* 295, no. 6 (2006): 643–54.

34   *Of the 1,001 substances:* "Agents Classified by the *IARC Monographs*, Volumes 1–118,"

IARC Monographs on the Evaluation of Carcinogenic Risks to Humans, April 13, 2017, http://monographs.iarc.fr/ENG/Classification/.

the organization has effectively lumped together: Ibid. (Search list of classifications.)

3. EGGS

42 *we need cholesterol:* National Cholesterol Education Program, "What Is Cholesterol?," in *Third Report of the National Cholesterol Education Program (NCEP) Expert Panel on Detection, Evaluation, and Treatment of High Blood Cholesterol in Adults (Adult Treatment Panel III): Final Report* (National Institutes of Health, National Heart, Lung, and Blood Institute, September 2002), https://www.nhlbi.nih.gov/sites/www.nhlbi.nih.gov/files/Circulation-2002-ATP-III-Final-Report-PDF-3143.pdf.

43 *calls to begin screening children:* "Expert Panel on Integrated Guidelines for Cardiovascular Health and Risk Reduction in Children and Adolescents: Summary Report," *Pediatrics* 128, suppl. 5 (2011): S213–56.

with kids once we test them: T. B. Newman, M. J. Pletcher, and S. B. Hulley, "Overly Aggressive New Guidelines for Lipid Screening in Children: Evidence of a Broken Process," *Pediatrics* 130, no. 2 (2012): 349–52.

44 *a 2004 study randomized:* K. L. Herron, I. E. Lofgren, M. Sharman, J. S. Volek, and M. L. Fernandez, "High Intake of Cholesterol Results in Less Atherogenic Low-Density Lipoprotein Particles in Men and Women Independent of Response Classification," *Metabolism: Clinical and Experimental* 53, no. 6 (2004): 823–30.

what we call "hyporesponders": M. L. Fernandez, "Dietary Cholesterol Provided by Eggs and Plasma Lipoproteins in Healthy Populations," *Current Opinion in Clinical Nutrition and Metabolic Care* 9, no. 1 (2006): 8–12.

45 *systematic review of studies:* J. D. Griffin and A. H. Lichtenstein, "Dietary Cholesterol and Plasma Lipoprotein Profiles: Randomized-Controlled Trials," *Current Nutrition Reports* 2, no. 4 (2013): 274–82.

ran the numbers on eggs and cholesterol: J. W. Vaupel and J. D. Graham, "Egg in Your Bier?," *Public Interest* (Winter 1980): 3–17.

46 *the committee published a report:* "Scientific Report of the 2015 Dietary Guidelines Advisory Committee" (U.S. Department of Agriculture and U.S. Department of Health and Human Services, first print, February 2015), https://health.gov/dietaryguidelines/2015-scientific-report/PDFs/Scientific-Report-of-the-2015-Dietary-Guidelines-Advisory-Committee.pdf.

released the updated guidelines in 2015: U.S. Department of Health and Human Services and U.S. Department of Agriculture, *2015–2020 Dietary Guidelines for Americans,* 8th ed. (December 2015), https://health.gov/dietaryguidelines/2015/guidelines/.

47 *you have to take "special care":* "Salmonella and Eggs," Centers for Disease Control and Prevention, https://www.cdc.gov/features/salmonellaeggs/.

48 *Decades ago, the threat of contracting:* Paul Patterson, "Egg Quality Assurance Programs," *New York Times,* updated August 25, 2010, https://www.nytimes.com/roomfordebate/2010/8/24/why-eggs-became-a-salmonella-hazard/egg-quality-assurance-programs.

Studies predict that 94%: B. K. Hope, R. Baker, E. D. Edel, A. T. Hogue, W. D. Schlosser, R. Whiting, et al., "An Overview of the *Salmonella enteritidis* Assessment for Shell Eggs and Egg Products," *Risk Analysis* 22, no. 2 (2002): 203–18.

4. SALT

52   *Research shows that it can even improve:* Institute of Medicine, Committee on Strategies to Reduce Sodium Intake, "Taste and Flavor Roles of Sodium in Foods: A Unique Challenge to Reducing Sodium Intake," in *Strategies to Reduce Sodium Intake in the United States,* ed. J. E. Henney, C. L. Taylor, and C. S. Boon (Washington, DC: National Academies Press, 2010), https://www.ncbi.nlm.nih.gov/books/NBK50958/.

54   *the first connection between salt consumption:* G. MacGregor and H. E. De Wardener, *Salt, Diet and Health: Neptune's Poisoned Chalice; The Origins of High Blood Pressure* (Cambridge: Cambridge University Press, 1998), xi.

        how much the subjects were eating: W. C. Roberts, "Facts and Ideas from Anywhere," editorial, *Proceedings (Baylor University Medical Center)* 14, no. 3 (2001): 314–22.

55   *a researcher named Walter Kempner:* MacGregor and De Wardener, *Salt, Diet and Health,* xi.

        more than 100,000 people in eighteen countries: A. Mente, M. J. O'Donnell, S. Rangarajan, M. J. McQueen, P. Poirier, A. Wielgosz, et al., "Association of Urinary Sodium and Potassium Excretion with Blood Pressure," *New England Journal of Medicine* 371, no. 7 (2014): 601–11.

56   *a significantly higher chance of death:* M. O'Donnell, A. Mente, S. Rangarajan, M. J. McQueen, X. Wang, L. Liu, et al., "Urinary Sodium and Potassium Excretion, Mortality, and Cardiovascular Events," *New England Journal of Medicine* 371, no. 7 (2014): 612–23.

        the Institute of Medicine assessed the evidence: Institute of Medicine, Committee on the Consequences of Sodium Reduction in the Population, *Sodium Intake in Populations: Assessment of Evidence,* ed. B. L. Strom, A. L. Yaktine, and M. Oria (Washington, DC: National Academies Press, 2013).

57   *followed 3,681 people over almost a decade:* K. Stolarz-Skrzypek, T. Kuznetsova, L. Thijs, V. Tikhonoff, J. Seidlerova, T. Richart, et al., "Fatal and Nonfatal Outcomes, Incidence of Hypertension, and Blood Pressure Changes in Relation to Urinary Sodium Excretion," *JAMA* 305, no. 17 (2011): 1777–85.

        A recent meta-analysis makes this point: A. Mente, M. O'Donnell, S. Rangarajan, G. Dagenais, S. Lear, M. McQueen, et al., "Associations of Urinary Sodium Excretion with Cardiovascular Events in Individuals with and Without Hypertension: A Pooled Analysis of Data from Four Studies," *Lancet* 388, no. 10043 (2016): 465–75.

59   *continue to insist that Americans:* U.S. Department of Health and Human Services and U.S. Department of Agriculture, *2015–2020 Dietary Guidelines.*

60   *slice of American cheese:* Centers for Disease Control and Prevention, "Get the Facts: Sources of Sodium in Your Diet" (Atlanta, April 2016), https://www.cdc.gov/salt/pdfs/sources_of_sodium.pdf.

        keeps a running tab: "Xtreme Eating 2016," Center for Science in the Public Interest, https://cspinet.org/eating-healthy/foods-avoid/xtreme2016.

61   *than the lunches provided by the school:* M. L. Caruso and K. W. Cullen, "Quality and

Cost of Student Lunches Brought from Home," *JAMA Pediatrics* 169, no. 1 (2015): 86–90.

without much damage to their bottom line: A. A. Patel, N. V. Lopez, H. T. Lawless, V. Njike, M. Beleche, and D. L. Katz, "Reducing Calories, Fat, Saturated Fat, and Sodium in Restaurant Menu Items: Effects on Consumer Acceptance," *Obesity* 24 (2016): 2497–2508.

62   *95% of people in eighteen countries:* Mente et al., "Associations of Urinary Sodium Excretion."

63   *one-third of adults have high blood pressure:* U.S. Food and Drug Administration, "FDA Issues Draft Guidance to Food Industry for Voluntarily Reducing Sodium in Processed and Commercially Prepared Food," press release, June 1, 2016.

5. GLUTEN

66   *if you are "gluten sensitive":* A. Sapone, J. C. Bai, C. Ciacci, J. Dolinsek, P. H. Green, M. Hadjivassiliou, et al., "Spectrum of Gluten-Related Disorders: Consensus on New Nomenclature and Classification," *BMC Medicine* 10, no. 1 (2012): 1–12.

67   *In Europe:* B. I. Nwaru, L. Hickstein, S. S. Panesar, G. Roberts, A. Muraro, and A. Sheikh, "Prevalence of Common Food Allergies in Europe: A Systematic Review and Meta-analysis," *Allergy* 69, no. 8 (2014): 992–1007

       In Asia: A. J. Lee, M. Thalayasingam, and B. W. Lee, "Food Allergy in Asia: How Does It Compare?," *Asia Pacific Allergy* 3, no. 1 (2013): 3–14.

       In the United States: C. A. Keet, E. C. Matsui, G. Dhillon, P. Lenehan, M. Paterakis, and R. A. Wood, "The Natural History of Wheat Allergy," *Annals of Allergy, Asthma & Immunology* 102, no. 5 (2009): 410–15.

69   *the prevalence of celiac disease in the United States:* A. Rubio-Tapia, J. F. Ludvigsson, T. L. Brantner, J. A. Murray, and J. E. Everhart, "The Prevalence of Celiac Disease in the United States," *American Journal of Gastroenterology* 107, no. 10 (2012): 1538–44.

       study published in the Journal of General Internal Medicine: R. D. Zipser, M. Farid, D. Baisch, B. Patel, and D. Patel, "Physician Awareness of Celiac Disease," *Journal of General Internal Medicine* 20, no. 7 (2005): 644–46.

70   *four times as likely to have celiac disease:* A. C. Ford, W. D. Chey, N. J. Talley, A. Malhotra, B. R. Spiegel, and P. Moayyedi, "Yield of Diagnostic Tests for Celiac Disease in Individuals with Symptoms Suggestive of Irritable Bowel Syndrome: Systematic Review and Meta-analysis," *Archives of Internal Medicine* 169, no. 7 (2009): 651–58.

       treated for iron and folate deficiencies: M. R. Howard, A. J. Turnbull, P. Morley, P. Hollier, R. Webb, and A. Clarke, "A Prospective Study of the Prevalence of Undiagnosed Coeliac Disease in Laboratory Defined Iron and Folate Deficiency," *Journal of Clinical Pathology* 55, no. 10 (2002): 754–57.

       a child who was diagnosed with autism: S. J. Genuis and T. P. Bouchard, "Celiac Disease Presenting as Autism," *Journal of Child Neurology* 25, no. 1 (2010): 114–19.

       U.S. Preventive Services Task Force: U.S. Preventive Services Task Force, "Draft Recommendation Statement: Celiac Disease; Screening" (May 30, 2016), https://www.uspreventiveservicestaskforce.org/Page/Document/draft-recommendation-statement150/celiac-disease-screening.

71   *study published in the* American Journal of Gastroenterology: J. R. Biesiekierski, E. D. Newnham, P. M. Irving, J. S. Barrett, M. Haines, J. D. Doecke, et al., "Gluten Causes Gastrointestinal Symptoms in Subjects Without Celiac Disease: A Double-Blind Randomized Placebo-Controlled Trial," *American Journal of Gastroenterology* 106, no. 3 (2011): 508–14.

     David Perlmutter's Grain Brain: D. Perlmutter with K. Loberg, *Grain Brain: The Surprising Truth About Wheat, Carbs, and Sugar — Your Brain's Silent Killers* (New York: Little, Brown, 2013), x.

72   *wheat breeding has not led:* D. D. Kasarda, "Can an Increase in Celiac Disease Be Attributed to an Increase in the Gluten Content of Wheat as a Consequence of Wheat Breeding?," *Journal of Agricultural and Food Chemistry* 61, no. 6 (2013): 1155–59.

     annual intake of wheat flour: "Wheat's Role in the U.S. Diet," U.S. Department of Agriculture, Economic Research Service, last updated October 26, 2016, https://www.ers. usda.gov/topics/crops/wheat/wheats-role-in-the-us-diet/.

     In 2014, it was estimated: Stephanie Strom, "A Big Bet on Gluten-Free," Business Day, *New York Times,* February 17, 2014, https://www.nytimes.com/2014/02/18/business/food-industry-wagers-big-on-gluten-free.html.

     a better study to confirm their findings: J. R. Biesiekierski, S. L. Peters, E. D. Newnham, O. Rosella, J. G. Muir, and P. R. Gibson, "No Effects of Gluten in Patients with Self-Reported Non-celiac Gluten Sensitivity After Dietary Reduction of Fermentable, Poorly Absorbed, Short-Chain Carbohydrates," *Gastroenterology* 145, no. 2 (2013): 320–28.e1–3.

73   *study published in 2014:* J. R. Biesiekierski, E. D. Newnham, S. J. Shepherd, J. G. Muir, and P. R. Gibson, "Characterization of Adults with a Self-Diagnosis of Nonceliac Gluten Sensitivity," *Nutrition in Clinical Practice* 29, no. 4 (2014): 504–9.

74   *study published in 2006:* W. Dickey and N. Kearney, "Overweight in Celiac Disease: Prevalence, Clinical Characteristics, and Effect of a Gluten-Free Diet," *American Journal of Gastroenterology* 101, no. 10 (2006): 2356–59.

     who were overweight almost doubled: E. Valletta, M. Fornaro, M. Cipolli, S. Conte, F. Bissolo, and C. Danchielli, "Celiac Disease and Obesity: Need for Nutritional Follow-Up After Diagnosis," *European Journal of Clinical Nutrition* 64, no. 11 (2010): 1371–72.

75   *article in the* Wall Street Journal: Julie Jargon, "The Gluten-Free Craze: Is It Healthy?," *Wall Street Journal,* June 22, 2014, http://online.wsj.com/articles/how-we-eat-the-gluten-free-craze-is-it-healthy-1403491041.

     study following thousands of health professionals: B. Lebwohl, Y. Cao, G. Zong, F. B. Hu, P.H.R. Green, A. I. Neugut, et al., "Long Term Gluten Consumption in Adults Without Celiac Disease and Risk of Coronary Heart Disease: Prospective Cohort Study," *BMJ* 357 (2017): j1892.

     lead to deficiencies in nutrients: D. Wild, G. G. Robins, V. J. Burley, and P. D. Howdle, "Evidence of High Sugar Intake, and Low Fibre and Mineral Intake, in the Gluten-Free Diet," *Alimentary Pharmacology & Therapeutics* 32, no. 4 (2010): 573–81.

76   *the nocebo effect with respect to pain:* G. L. Petersen, N. B. Finnerup, L. Colloca, M. Amanzio, D. D. Price, T. S. Jensen, et al., "The Magnitude of Nocebo Effects in Pain: A Meta-analysis," *Pain* 155, no. 8 (2014): 1426–34.

77   *underwent laboratory testing for celiac disease:* H. S. Kim, K. G. Patel, E. Orosz, N. Kothari, M. F. Demyen, N. Pyrsopoulos, et al., "Time Trends in the Prevalence of Celiac

Disease and Gluten-Free Diet in the US Population: Results from the National Health and Nutrition Examination Surveys 2009–2014," *JAMA Internal Medicine* 176, no. 11 (2016): 1716–17.

the prevalence of strict gluten-free diets: Ibid.

78   *the prevalence varies in different populations:* U. Volta, G. Caio, F. Tovoli, and R. De Giorgio, "Non-celiac Gluten Sensitivity: Questions Still to Be Answered Despite Increasing Awareness," *Cellular & Molecular Immunology* 10, no. 5 (2013): 383–92.

nowhere near the one-third of consumers: Nancy Shute, "Gluten Goodbye: One-Third of Americans Say They're Trying to Shun It," Eating and Health, *The Salt: What's on Your Plate,* NPR, March 9, 2013, http://www.npr.org/sections/the salt/2013/03/09/173840841/gluten-goodbye-one-third-of-americans-say-theyre-try ing-to-shun-it.

Sales of products with gluten-free labels: Jargon, "The Gluten-Free Craze."

6. GMOs

79   *hundreds of millions of people would starve:* P. R. Ehrlich, *The Population Bomb* (New York: Ballantine, 1968).

80   *He was massively successful:* D. Biello, "Norman Borlaug: Wheat Breeder Who Averted Famine with a 'Green Revolution,'" *News Blog, Scientific American,* September 14, 2009, https://blogs.scientificamerican.com/news-blog/norman-borlaug-wheat-breeder-who-av-2009-09-14/.

six times more wheat than they had been: "Genetically Modified Organisms (GMOs)," *Nature News,* n.d., http://www.nature.com/scitable/spotlight/gmos-6978241.

81   *the Guardian could publish a blog post:* J. Vidal, "Norman Borlaug: Humanitarian Hero or Menace to Society?," *Poverty Matters* (blog), *Guardian,* April 1, 2014, https://www.theguardian.com/global-development/poverty-matters/2014/apr/01/norman-bor laug-humanitarian-hero-menace-society.

83   *GMOs are also really common:* "Recent Trends in GE Adoption," U.S. Department of Agriculture, Economic Research Service, last updated November 3, 2016, https://www.ers.usda.gov/data-products/adoption-of-genetically-engineered-crops-in-the-us/recent-trends-in-ge-adoption.aspx.

84   *report reviewing all the available evidence:* National Research Council and Institute of Medicine, *Safety of Genetically Engineered Foods: Approaches to Assessing Unintended Health Effects* (Washington, DC: National Academies Press, 2004).

The European Union conducted: European Commission, "A Decade of EU-Funded GMO Research (2001–2010)" (Luxembourg: Publication Office of the European Union, 2010).

85   *Pew poll in 2015:* Cary Funk, "5 Key Findings on What Americans and Scientists Think About Science," *Fact Tank,* Pew Research Center, January 29, 2015, http://www.pewre search.org/fact-tank/2015/01/29/5-key-findings-science/.

In Europe, regulations regarding their use: S. Wunderlich and K. A. Gatto, "Consumer Perception of Genetically Modified Organisms and Sources of Information," *Advances in Nutrition* 6, no. 6 (2015): 842–51.

86   *This happened in Oregon:* Dan Charles, "GMO Wheat Found in Oregon Field: How Did

It Get There?," Producers, *The Salt: What's on Your Plate,* NPR, May 30, 2013, http://www.npr.org/blogs/thesalt/2013/05/30/187103955/gmo-wheat-found-in-oregon-field-howd-it-get-there.

87   *GENera published a systematic review:* A. Nicolia, A. Manzo, F. Veronesi, and D. Rosellini, "An Overview of the Last 10 Years of Genetically Engineered Crop Safety Research," *Critical Reviews in Biotechnology* 34, no. 1 (2014): 77–88.

It was then shown: Allison Aubrey, "Class-Action Suit Alleges Chipotle's GMO-Free Campaign Is Deceptive," Food for Thought, *Salt: What's on Your Plate,* NPR, September 2, 2015, http://www.npr.org/sections/thesalt/2015/09/02/436673039/class-action-suit-alleges-chipotles-gmo-free-campaign-is-deceptive.

88   *more likely to lead to unintended consequences:* Institute of Medicine, Committee on Identifying and Assessing Unintended Effects of Genetically Engineered Foods on Human Health, *Safety of Genetically Engineered Foods: Approaches to Assessing Unintended Health Effects* (Washington, DC: National Academies Press, 2004), xvii.

91   *most comprehensive review of GMO safety:* National Academies of Sciences, Engineering, and Medicine, *Genetically Engineered Crops: Experiences and Prospects* (Washington, DC: National Academies Press, 2016).

7. ALCOHOL

96   *epidemiologic study published in 1990:* P. Boffetta and L. Garfinkel, "Alcohol Drinking and Mortality Among Men Enrolled in an American Cancer Society Prospective Study," *Epidemiology* 1, no. 5 (1990): 342–48.

97   *A 2004 observational study:* M. Gronbaek, D. Johansen, U. Becker, H. O. Hein, P. Schnohr, G. Jensen, et al., "Changes in Alcohol Intake and Mortality: A Longitudinal Population-Based Study," *Epidemiology* 15, no. 2 (2004): 222–28.

consistent across a number of studies: R. Doll, R. Peto, E. Hall, K. Wheatley, and R. Gray, "Mortality in Relation to Consumption of Alcohol: 13 Years' Observations on Male British Doctors," *BMJ* 309, no. 6959 (1994): 911–18; M. Gronbaek, U. Becker, D. Johansen, A. Gottschau, P. Schnohr, H. O. Hein, et al., "Type of Alcohol Consumed and Mortality from All Causes, Coronary Heart Disease, and Cancer," *Annals of Internal Medicine* 133, no. 6 (2000): 411–19.

published in the gloomily titled journal: C. J. Holahan, K. K. Schutte, P. L. Brennan, C. K. Holahan, B. S. Moos, and R. H. Moos, "Late-Life Alcohol Consumption and 20-Year Mortality," *Alcoholism: Clinical and Experimental Research* 34, no. 11 (2010): 1961–71.

almost all of the major benefits of drinking: K. J. Mukamal, K. M. Conigrave, M. A. Mittleman, C.A.J. Camargo, M. J. Stampfer, W. C. Willett, et al., "Roles of Drinking Pattern and Type of Alcohol Consumed in Coronary Heart Disease in Men," *New England Journal of Medicine* 348, no. 2 (2003): 109–18.

98   *still obtaining this protective effect:* M. J. Thun, R. Peto, A. D. Lopez, J. H. Monaco, S. J. Henley, C.W.J. Heath, et al., "Alcohol Consumption and Mortality Among Middle-Aged and Elderly U.S. Adults," *New England Journal of Medicine* 337, no. 24 (1997): 1705–14.

A 2007 study involving the Women's Health Study cohort: S. M. Zhang, I.-M. Lee, J. E. Manson, N. R. Cook, W. C. Willett, and J. E. Buring, "Alcohol Consumption and Breast

Cancer Risk in the Women's Health Study," *American Journal of Epidemiology* 165, no. 6 (2007): 667–76.

a 2014 systematic review of research: C. Scoccianti, B. Lauby-Secretan, P. Y. Bello, V. Chajes, and I. Romieu, "Female Breast Cancer and Alcohol Consumption: A Review of the Literature," *American Journal of Preventive Medicine* 46, no. 3 (2014): S16–25.

meta-analysis of studies: S. Cai, Y. Li, Y. Ding, K. Chen, and M. Jin, "Alcohol Drinking and the Risk of Colorectal Cancer Death: A Meta-analysis," *European Journal of Cancer Prevention* 23, no. 6 (2014): 532–39.

bladder cancer: C. Pelucchi, C. Galeone, I. Tramacere, V. Bagnardi, E. Negri, F. Islami, et al., "Alcohol Drinking and Bladder Cancer Risk: A Meta-analysis," *Annals of Oncology* 23, no. 6 (2012): 1586–93.

ovarian cancer: M. Rota, E. Pasquali, L. Scotti, C. Pelucchi, I. Tramacere, F. Islami, et al., "Alcohol Drinking and Epithelial Ovarian Cancer Risk. A Systematic Review and Meta-analysis," *Gynecologic Oncology* 125, no. 3 (2012): 758–63.

heavy drinking was detrimental: M. Jin, S. Cai, J. Guo, Y. Zhu, M. Li, Y. Yu, et al., "Alcohol Drinking and All Cancer Mortality: A Meta-analysis," *Annals of Oncology* 24, no. 3 (2013): 807–16.

cohort of about 6,000 people: A. Britton, A. Singh-Manoux, and M. Marmot, "Alcohol Consumption and Cognitive Function in the Whitehall II Study," *American Journal of Epidemiology* 160, no. 3 (2004): 240–47.

99 *A 2004 systematic review:* A. A. Howard, J. H. Arnsten, and M. N. Gourevitch, "Effect of Alcohol Consumption on Diabetes Mellitus: A Systematic Review," *Annals of Internal Medicine* 140, no. 3 (2004): 211–19.

In 2015, such a trial was published: Y. Gepner, R. Golan, I. Harman-Boehm, Y. Henkin, D. Schwarzfuchs, I. Shelef, et al., "Effects of Initiating Moderate Alcohol Intake on Cardiometabolic Risk in Adults with Type 2 Diabetes: A 2-Year Randomized, Controlled Trial," *Annals of Internal Medicine* 163, no. 8 (2015): 569–79.

another analysis of the same study: Y. Gepner, Y. Henkin, D. Schwarzfuchs, R. Golan, R. Durst, I. Shelef, et al., "Differential Effect of Initiating Moderate Red Wine Consumption on 24-h Blood Pressure by Alcohol Dehydrogenase Genotypes: Randomized Trial in Type 2 Diabetes," *American Journal of Hypertension* 29, no. 4 (2016): 476–83.

100 *small but significant increase in blood pressure:* C. B. McFadden, C. M. Brensinger, J. A. Berlin, and R. R. Townsend, "Systemic Review of the Effect of Daily Alcohol Intake on Blood Pressure," *American Journal of Hypertension* 18, no. 2 (2005): 276–86.

shorter-term trial looking at red wine: D. W. Droste, C. Iliescu, M. Vaillant, M. Gantenbein, N. De Bremaeker, C. Lieunard, et al., "A Daily Glass of Red Wine and Lifestyle Changes Do Not Affect Arterial Blood Pressure and Heart Rate in Patients with Carotid Arteriosclerosis After 4 and 20 Weeks," *Cerebrovascular Diseases Extra* 3, no. 1 (2013): 121–29.

improved cholesterol levels: D. W. Droste, C. Iliescu, M. Vaillant, M. Gantenbein, N. De Bremaeker, C. Lieunard, et al., "A Daily Glass of Red Wine Associated with Lifestyle Changes Independently Improves Blood Lipids in Patients with Carotid Arteriosclerosis: Results from a Randomized Controlled Trial," *Nutrition Journal* 12, no. 1 (2013): 147.

a 2011 meta-analysis: S. E. Brien, P. E. Ronksley, B. J. Turner, K. J. Mukamal, and W. A. Ghali, "Effect of Alcohol Consumption on Biological Markers Associated with Risk of

Coronary Heart Disease: Systematic Review and Meta-analysis of Interventional Studies," *BMJ* 342 (2011): d636.

101   *gains in cardiovascular disease:* I. R. White, D. R. Altmann, and K. Nanchahal, "Alcohol Consumption and Mortality: Modelling Risks for Men and Women at Different Ages," *BMJ* 325, no. 7357 (2002): 191.

  The most recent report: U.S. Department of Health and Human Services and U.S. Department of Agriculture, *2015–2020 Dietary Guidelines for Americans*, 8th ed. (December 2015), appendix 9, https://health.gov/dietaryguidelines/2015/guidelines/appen dix-9/.

  "a little alcohol may not be good for you after all": S. Begley, "A Little Alcohol May Not Be Good for You After All," *STAT*, March 22, 2016, https://www.statnews.com/2016/03/22/alcohol-longevity-benefit-challenged.

102   *an updated systematic review:* T. Stockwell, J. Zhao, S. Panwar, A. Roemer, T. Naimi, and T. Chikritzhs, "Do 'Moderate' Drinkers Have Reduced Mortality Risk? A Systematic Review and Meta-analysis of Alcohol Consumption and All-Cause Mortality," *Journal of Studies on Alcohol and Drugs* 77, no. 2 (2016): 185–98.

103   *one study I discussed earlier:* Holahan et al., "Late-Life Alcohol Consumption."

  looked at mortality from a variety: P. E. Ronksley, S. E. Brien, B. J. Turner, K. J. Mukamal, and W. A. Ghali, "Association of Alcohol Consumption with Selected Cardiovascular Disease Outcomes: A Systematic Review and Meta-analysis," *BMJ* 342 (2011): d671.

104   *better cognitive function:* Britton, Singh-Manoux, and Marmot, "Alcohol Consumption and Cognitive Function."

  lower rates of diabetes: Howard, Arnsten, and Gourevitch, "Effect of Alcohol Consumption on Diabetes Mellitus."

  improved blood lipids: Droste et al., "A Daily Glass of Red Wine Associated with Lifestyle Changes Independently Improves Blood Lipids."

  stave off diabetes: Gepner, Golan, Harman-Boehm, et al., "Effects of Initiating Moderate Alcohol Intake on Cardiometabolic Risk in Adults with Type 2 Diabetes."

  improve blood pressure: Gepner, Henkin, Schwarzfuchs, et al., "Differential Effect of Initiating Moderate Red Wine Consumption on 24-h Blood Pressure."

  meta-analysis of sixty-three controlled trials: Brien et al., "Effect of Alcohol Consumption on Biological Markers Associated with Risk of Coronary Heart Disease."

105   *differences between men and women:* Anastasia Toufexis, "Why Men Can Outdrink Women," *Time*, June 24, 2001, http://content.time.com/time/magazine/article/0,9171,153672,00.html.

  Philip J. Cook used data: P. J. Cook, *Paying the Tab: The Economics of Alcohol Policy* (Princeton, NJ: Princeton University Press; 2007), xiii.

107   *A 2012 Centers for Disease Control and Prevention report:* Centers for Disease Control and Prevention, "Vital Signs: Binge Drinking Prevalence, Frequency, and Intensity Among Adults — United States, 2010," *Morbidity and Mortality Weekly Report* 61, no. 1 (2012): 14.

108   *study in the journal* Pediatrics: L. A. Teplin, J. A. Jakubowski, K. M. Abram, N. D. Olson, M. L. Stokes, and L. J. Welty, "Firearm Homicide and Other Causes of Death in Delinquents: A 16-Year Prospective Study," *Pediatrics* 134, no. 1 (2014): 66–73.

  A 2014 prospective study: R. C. Shorey, G. L. Stuart, T. M. Moore, and J. K. McNulty, "The Temporal Relationship Between Alcohol, Marijuana, Angry Affect, and Dating Violence Perpetration: A Daily Diary Study with Female College Students," *Psychology of Addictive Behaviors* 28, no. 2 (2014): 516–23.

A 2016 report on colleges and drinking: "Fall Semester — a Time for Parents to Discuss the Risks of College Drinking," National Institute on Alcohol Abuse and Alcoholism, updated October 2016, https://pubs.niaaa.nih.gov/publications/CollegeFactSheet/back_to_collegeFact.htm.

About 600,000 are injured: A. White and R. Hingson, "The Burden of Alcohol Use: Excessive Alcohol Consumption and Related Consequences Among College Students," *Alcohol Research: Current Reviews* 35, no. 2 (2014): 201.

only a small step to addiction: C. Lopez-Quintero, J. Perez de los Cobos, D. S. Hasin, M. Okuda, S. Wang, B. F. Grant, et al., "Probability and Predictors of Transition from First Use to Dependence on Nicotine, Alcohol, Cannabis, and Cocaine: Results of the National Epidemiologic Survey on Alcohol and Related Conditions (NESARC)," *Drug and Alcohol Dependence* 115, nos. 1–2 (2011): 120–30.

It ranked drugs: D. J. Nutt, L. A. King, and L. D. Phillips, "Drug Harms in the UK: A Multicriteria Decision Analysis," *Lancet* 376, no. 9752 (2010): 1558–65.

109   *Most of the research that links:* C. O'Leary, S. R. Zubrick, C. L. Taylor, G. Dixon, and C. Bower, "Prenatal Alcohol Exposure and Language Delay in 2-Year-Old Children: The Importance of Dose and Timing on Risk," *Pediatrics* 123, no. 2 (2009): 547–54.

Some studies show that more than twice: S. Popova, S. Lange, C. Probst, G. Gmel, and J. Rehm, "Estimation of National, Regional, and Global Prevalence of Alcohol Use During Pregnancy and Fetal Alcohol Syndrome: A Systematic Review and Meta-analysis," *Lancet Global Health* 5, no. 3 (2017): e290–99.

a large cohort study in Denmark: A. Skogerbo, U. S. Kesmodel, T. Wimberley, H. Stovring, J. Bertrand, N. I. Landro, et al., "The Effects of Low to Moderate Alcohol Consumption and Binge Drinking in Early Pregnancy on Executive Function in 5-Year-Old Children," *BJOG* 119, no. 10 (2012): 1201–10.

110   *one of the most cited studies on this subject:* B. Sood, V. Delaney-Black, C. Covington, B. Nordstrom-Klee, J. Ager, T. Templin, et al., "Prenatal Alcohol Exposure and Childhood Behavior at Age 6 to 7 Years: I. Dose-Response Effect," *Pediatrics* 108, no. 2 (2001): E34.

study published in 2010 surveyed obstetricians: B. L. Anderson, E. P. Dang, R. L. Floyd, R. Sokol, J. Mahoney, and J. Schulkin, "Knowledge, Opinions, and Practice Patterns of Obstetrician-Gynecologists Regarding Their Patients' Use of Alcohol," *Journal of Addiction Medicine* 4, no. 2 (2010): 114–21.

111   *Expecting Better:* E. Oster, *Expecting Better: Why the Conventional Wisdom Is Wrong — and What You Really Need to Know* (New York: Penguin, 2013), xxii.

112   *If alcohol is consumed:* U.S. Department of Health and Human Services and U.S. Department of Agriculture, *2015–2020 Dietary Guidelines for Americans,* appendix 9.

8. COFFEE

114   *Coffee has long had a reputation:* J. Stromberg, "It's a Myth: There's No Evidence That Coffee Stunts Kids' Growth," Smithsonian.com, December 20, 2013.

116   *a 1993 study that reviewed:* L. K. Massey and S. J. Whiting, "Caffeine, Urinary Calcium, Calcium Metabolism and Bone," *Journal of Nutrition* 123, no. 9 (1993): 1611–14.

Another study, this one in 2002: R. P. Heaney, "Effects of Caffeine on Bone and the Calcium Economy," *Food and Chemical Toxicology* 40, no. 9 (2002): 1263–70.

A 1998 study followed: T. Lloyd, N. J. Rollings, K. Kieselhorst, D. F. Eggli, and E. Mauger, "Dietary Caffeine Intake Is Not Correlated with Adolescent Bone Gain," *Journal of the American College of Nutrition* 17, no. 5 (1998): 454–57.

117 *Another study from two years earlier:* P. T. Packard and R. R. Recker, "Caffeine Does Not Affect the Rate of Gain in Spine Bone in Young Women," *Osteoporosis International* 6, no. 2 (1996): 149–52.

Combining the results of sixteen trials: Y. Zhang, A. Coca, D. J. Casa, J. Antonio, J. M. Green, and P. A. Bishop, "Caffeine and Diuresis During Rest and Exercise: A Meta-analysis," *Journal of Science and Medicine in Sport* 18, no. 5 (2015): 569–74.

118 *studies show that tea:* C. H. Ruxton and V. A. Hart, "Black Tea Is Not Significantly Different from Water in the Maintenance of Normal Hydration in Human Subjects: Results from a Randomised Controlled Trial," *British Journal of Nutrition* 106, no. 4 (2011): 588–95.

Carbonated beverages with caffeine: A. C. Grandjean, K. J. Reimers, K. E. Bannick, and M. C. Haven, "The Effect of Caffeinated, Non-caffeinated, Caloric and Non-caloric Beverages on Hydration," *Journal of the American College of Nutrition* 19, no. 5 (2000): 591–600.

119 *In 2015, I agreed to write:* Aaron E. Carroll, "More Consensus on Coffee's Effect on Health Than You Might Think," Upshot (blog), *New York Times,* May 11, 2015, https://www.nytimes.com/2015/05/12/upshot/more-consensus-on-coffees-benefits-than-you-might-think.html.

a 2014 systematic review and meta-analysis: M. Ding, S. N. Bhupathiraju, A. Satija, R. M. van Dam, and F. B. Hu, "Long-Term Coffee Consumption and Risk of Cardiovascular Disease: A Systematic Review and a Dose-Response Meta-analysis of Prospective Cohort Studies," *Circulation* 129, no. 6 (2014): 643–59.

120 *meta-analysis looking at how coffee consumption:* S. C. Larsson and N. Orsini, "Coffee Consumption and Risk of Stroke: A Dose-Response Meta-analysis of Prospective Studies," *American Journal of Epidemiology* 174, no. 9 (2011): 993–1001.

meta-analysis published a year later: B. Kim, Y. Nam, J. Kim, H. Choi, and C. Won, "Coffee Consumption and Stroke Risk: A Meta-analysis of Epidemiologic Studies," *Korean Journal of Family Medicine* 33, no. 6 (2012): 356–65.

Another meta-analysis published the same year: E. Mostofsky, M. S. Rice, E. B. Levitan, and M. A. Mittleman, "Habitual Coffee Consumption and Risk of Heart Failure: A Dose-Response Meta-analysis," *Circulation: Heart Failure* 5, no. 4 (2012): 401–5.

121 *meta-analysis published in 2007:* S. C. Larsson and A. Wolk, "Coffee Consumption and Risk of Liver Cancer: A Meta-analysis," *Gastroenterology* 132, no. 5 (2007): 1740–45.

Two more-recent studies: L.-X. Sang, B. Chang, X.-H. Li, and M. Jiang, "Consumption of Coffee Associated with Reduced Risk of Liver Cancer: A Meta-analysis," *BMC Gastroenterology* 13, no. 1 (2013): 1–13; F. Bravi, C. Bosetti, A. Tavani, S. Gallus, and C. La Vecchia, "Coffee Reduces Risk for Hepatocellular Carcinoma: An Updated Meta-analysis," *Clinical Gastroenterology and Hepatology* 11, no. 11 (2013): 1413–21.e1.

meta-analyses looking at prostate cancer: C.-H. Park, S.-K. Myung, T.-Y. Kim, H. G. Seo, Y.-J. Jeon, Y. Kim, et al., "Coffee Consumption and Risk of Prostate Cancer: A Meta-analysis of Epidemiological Studies," *BJU International* 106, no. 6 (2010): 762–69; A.

Discacciati, N. Orsini, and A. Wolk, "Coffee Consumption and Risk of Nonaggressive, Aggressive and Fatal Prostate Cancer — A Dose-Response Meta-analysis," *Annals of Oncology* 25, no. 3 (2014): 584–91.

same holds true for breast cancer: W. Jiang, Y. Wu, and X. Jiang, "Coffee and Caffeine Intake and Breast Cancer Risk: An Updated Dose-Response Meta-analysis of 37 Published Studies," *Gynecologic Oncology* 129, no. 3 (2013): 620–29; N. Tang, B. Zhou, B. Wang, and R. Yu, "Coffee Consumption and Risk of Breast Cancer: A Metaanalysis," *American Journal of Obstetrics and Gynecology* 200, no. 3 (2009): 290.e1–9.

meta-analysis of studies on lung cancer: N. Tang, Y. Wu, J. Ma, B. Wang, and R. Yu, "Coffee Consumption and Risk of Lung Cancer: A Meta-analysis," *Lung Cancer* 67, no. 1 (2010): 17–22.

study looking at all cancers combined: X. Yu, Z. Bao, J. Zou, and J. Dong, "Coffee Consumption and Risk of Cancers: A Meta-analysis of Cohort Studies," *BMC Cancer* 11, no. 1 (2011): 1–11.

systematic review showed: S. Saab, D. Mallam, G. A. Cox, and M. J. Tong, "Impact of Coffee on Liver Diseases: A Systematic Review," *Liver International* 34, no. 4 (2014): 495–504.

122   *lower risk of Parkinson's disease:* H. Qi and S. Li, "Dose-Response Meta-analysis on Coffee, Tea and Caffeine Consumption with Risk of Parkinson's Disease," *Geriatrics & Gerontology International* 14, no. 2 (2014): 430–39.

lower cognitive decline in old age: L. Arab, F. Khan, and H. Lam, "Epidemiologic Evidence of a Relationship Between Tea, Coffee, or Caffeine Consumption and Cognitive Decline," *Advances in Nutrition* 4, no. 1 (2013): 115–22.

potential protective effect against Alzheimer's: C. Santos, J. Costa, J. Santos, A. Vaz-Carneiro, and N. Lunet, "Caffeine Intake and Dementia: Systematic Review and Meta-analysis," *Journal of Alzheimer's Disease* 20, suppl. 1 (2010): S187–204.

systematic review published in 2005: R. M. van Dam and F. B. Hu, "Coffee Consumption and Risk of Type 2 Diabetes: A Systematic Review," *JAMA* 294, no. 1 (2005): 97–104.

more recent study, published in 2014: M. Ding, S. N. Bhupathiraju, M. Chen, R. M. van Dam, and F. B Hu, "Caffeinated and Decaffeinated Coffee Consumption and Risk of Type 2 Diabetes: A Systematic Review and a Dose-Response Meta-analysis," *Diabetes Care* 37, no. 2 (2014): 569–86.

meta-analysis published in 2014: Y. Je and E. Giovannucci, "Coffee Consumption and Total Mortality: A Meta-analysis of Twenty Prospective Cohort Studies," *British Journal of Nutrition* 111, no. 7 (2014): 1162–73.

another, published in 2015: Y. Zhao, K. Wu, J. Zheng, R. Zuo, and D. Li, "Association of Coffee Drinking with All-Cause Mortality: A Systematic Review and Meta-analysis," *Public Health Nutrition* 18, no. 7 (2015): 1282–91.

The study on diabetes and coffee: Ding, Bhupathiraju, Chen, et al., "Caffeinated and Decaffeinated Coffee Consumption."

123   *A 2005 meta-analysis:* M. Noordzij, C. S. Uiterwaal, L. R. Arends, F. J. Kok, D. E. Grobbee, and J. M. Geleijnse, "Blood Pressure Response to Chronic Intake of Coffee and Caffeine: A Meta-analysis of Randomized Controlled Trials," *Journal of Hypertension* 23, no. 5 (2005): 921–28.

124   *A 2011 study found:* A. E. Mesas, L. M. Leon-Muñoz, F. Rodriguez-Artalejo, and E. Lopez-Garcia, "The Effect of Coffee on Blood Pressure and Cardiovascular Disease in Hy-

pertensive Individuals: A Systematic Review and Meta-analysis," *American Journal of Clinical Nutrition* 94, no. 4 (2011): 1113–26.

Finally, a 2012 meta-analysis: M. Steffen, C. Kuhle, D. Hensrud, P. J. Erwin, and M. H. Murad, "The Effect of Coffee Consumption on Blood Pressure and the Development of Hypertension: A Systematic Review and Meta-analysis," *Journal of Hypertension* 30, no. 12 (2012): 2245–54.

two studies have shown: L. Cai, D. Ma, Y. Zhang, Z. Liu, and P. Wang, "The Effect of Coffee Consumption on Serum Lipids: A Meta-analysis of Randomized Controlled Trials," *European Journal of Clinical Nutrition* 66, no. 8 (2012): 872–77; S. H. Jee, J. He, L. J. Appel, P. K. Whelton, I. Suh, and M. J. Klag, "Coffee Consumption and Serum Lipids: A Meta-analysis of Randomized Controlled Clinical Trials," *American Journal of Epidemiology* 153, no. 4 (2001): 353–62.

125   *coffee is not only okay:* U.S. Department of Health and Human Services and U.S. Department of Agriculture, *2015–2020 Dietary Guidelines for Americans,* 8th ed. (December 2015), https://health.gov/dietaryguidelines/2015/guidelines/.

caffeine consumption and risk of miscarriage: L. Fenster, A. E. Hubbard, S. H. Swan, G. C. Windham, K. Waller, R. A. Hiatt, et al., "Caffeinated Beverages, Decaffeinated Coffee, and Spontaneous Abortion," *Epidemiology* 8, no. 5 (1997): 515–23.

more likely to smoke cigarettes: L. Chen, E. M. Bell, M. L. Browne, C. M. Druschel, and P. A. Romitti, "Exploring Maternal Patterns of Dietary Caffeine Consumption Before Conception and During Pregnancy," *Maternal and Child Health Journal* 18, no. 10 (2014): 2446–55.

126   *one 2016 study:* G. M. Buck Louis, K. J. Sapra, E. F. Schisterman, C. D. Lynch, J. M. Maisog, K. L. Grantz, et al., "Lifestyle and Pregnancy Loss in a Contemporary Cohort of Women Recruited Before Conception: The LIFE Study," *Fertility and Sterility* 106, no. 1 (2016): 180–88.

a 2010 systematic review: J. D. Peck, A. Leviton, and L. D. Cowan, "A Review of the Epidemiologic Evidence Concerning the Reproductive Health Effects of Caffeine Consumption: A 2000–2009 Update," *Food and Chemical Toxicology* 48, no. 10 (2010): 2549–76.

one randomized controlled trial even found: S. Jahanfar and S. H. Jaafar, "Effects of Restricted Caffeine Intake by Mother on Fetal, Neonatal and Pregnancy Outcomes," *Cochrane Database of Systematic Reviews,* no. 6 (2015).

127   *the WHO reclassified coffee:* World Health Organization, International Agency for Research on Cancer, "IARC Monographs Evaluate Drinking Coffee, Maté, and Very Hot Beverages," press release, June 15, 2016, https://www.iarc.fr/en/media-centre/pr/2016/pdfs/pr244_E.pdf.

9. DIET SODA

129   *first piece I wrote on this subject:* A. E. Carroll, "The Evidence Supports Artificial Sweeteners over Sugar," *Upshot* (blog), *New York Times,* July 27, 2015, https://www.nytimes.com/2015/07/28/upshot/the-evidence-supports-artificial-sweeteners-over-sugar.html.

134   *stumbled upon a treasure trove of documents:* C. E. Kearns, L. A. Schmidt, and S. A. Glantz, "Sugar Industry and Coronary Heart Disease Research: A Historical Analysis of Internal Industry Documents," *JAMA Internal Medicine* 176, no. 11 (2016): 1680–85.
   Sugar Research Foundation sponsored: R. B. McGandy, D. M. Hegsted, and F. J. Stare, "Dietary Fats, Carbohydrates and Atherosclerotic Vascular Disease," pt. 1, *New England Journal of Medicine* 277, no. 4 (1967): 186–92; ibid., pt. 2, *New England Journal of Medicine* 277, no. 5 (1967): 245–47.

135   *the foundation told Hegsted:* Ibid.
   two-part report: Ibid.

136   *study published in 2014:* Q. Yang, Z. Zhang, E. W. Gregg, W. Flanders, R. Merritt, and F. B. Hu, "Added Sugar Intake and Cardiovascular Diseases Mortality Among US Adults," *JAMA Internal Medicine* 174, no. 4 (2014): 516–24.
   The accompanying editorial argued: L. A. Schmidt, "New Unsweetened Truths About Sugar," *JAMA Internal Medicine* 174, no. 4 (2014): 525–26.

137   *a study published in 2016:* R. H. Lustig, K. Mulligan, S. M. Noworolski, V. W. Tai, M. J. Wen, A. Erkin-Cakmak, et al., "Isocaloric Fructose Restriction and Metabolic Improvement in Children with Obesity and Metabolic Syndrome," *Obesity* 24, no. 2 (2016): 453–60.

138   *Centers for Disease Control and Prevention reports:* R. B. Ervin, B. K. Kit, M. D. Carroll, and C. L. Ogden, "Consumption of Added Sugar Among U.S. Children and Adolescents, 2005–2008" (National Center for Health Statistics, Data Brief No. 87, March 2012), https://www.cdc.gov/nchs/data/databriefs/db87.pdf.
   Adults are doing slightly better: R. B. Ervin and C. L. Ogden, "Consumption of Added Sugars Among U.S. Adults, 2005–2010" (National Center for Health Statistics, Data Brief No. 122, May 2013), https://www.cdc.gov/nchs/data/databriefs/db122.pdf.
   This consumption isn't distributed equally: C. L. Ogden, B. K. Kit, M. D. Carroll, and S. Park, "Consumption of Sugar Drinks in the United States, 2005–2008" (National Center for Health Statistics, Data Brief No. 71, August 2013), https://www.cdc.gov/nchs/data/databriefs/db71.pdf.
   examined thirty randomized controlled trials: L. Te Morenga, S. Mallard, and J. Mann, "Dietary Sugars and Body Weight: Systematic Review and Meta-analyses of Randomised Controlled Trials and Cohort Studies," *BMJ* 346 (2013): e7492.

139   *study published in 2013:* S. Basu, P. Yoffe, N. Hills, and R. H. Lustig, "The Relationship of Sugar to Population-Level Diabetes Prevalence: An Econometric Analysis of Repeated Cross-Sectional Data," *PLOS ONE* 8, no. 2 (2013): e57873.

141   *accompanied by the following warning:* "Artificial Sweeteners and Cancer," National Cancer Institute, reviewed August 5, 2009, https://www.cancer.gov/about-cancer/causes-prevention/risk/diet/artificial-sweeteners-fact-sheet.
   summary of the history of saccharin: M. R. Weihrauch and V. Diehl, "Artificial Sweeteners — Do They Bear a Carcinogenic Risk?," *Annals of Oncology* 15, no. 10 (2004): 1460–65.
   In only one of those studies: S. Fukushima, M. Arai, J. Nakanowatari, T. Hibino, M. Okuda, and N. Ito, "Differences in Susceptibility to Sodium Saccharin Among Various Strains of Rats and Other Animal Species," *Gann* 74, no. 1 (1983): 8–20.

143   *they get bladder cancer:* Weihrauch and Diehl, "Artificial Sweeteners."

Studies in humans in the UK, Denmark, Canada, and the United States: B. Armstrong and R. Doll, "Bladder Cancer Mortality in England and Wales in Relation to Cigarette Smoking and Saccharin Consumption," *British Journal of Preventive & Social Medicine* 28, no. 4 (1974): 233–40; O. M. Jensen and C. Kamby, "Intra-Uterine Exposure to Saccharin and Risk of Bladder Cancer in Man," *International Journal of Cancer* 29, no. 5 (1982): 507–9; H. A. Risch, J. D. Burch, A. B. Miller, G. B. Hill, R. Steele, and G. R. Howe, "Dietary Factors and the Incidence of Cancer of the Urinary Bladder," *American Journal of Epidemiology* 127, no. 6 (1988): 1179–91.

published in the Journal of Neuropathology & Experimental Neurology: J. W. Olney, N. B. Farber, E. Spitznagel, and L. N. Robins, "Increasing Brain Tumor Rates: Is There a Link to Aspartame?," *Journal of Neuropathology & Experimental Neurology* 55, no. 11 (1996): 1115–23.

144   *a case-control study of children:* J. G. Gurney, J. M. Pogoda, E. A. Holly, S. S. Hecht, and S. Preston-Martin, "Aspartame Consumption in Relation to Childhood Brain Tumor Risk: Results from a Case-Control Study," *Journal of the National Cancer Institute* 89, no. 14 (1997): 1072–74.

a cohort study of more than 450,000 adults: U. Lim, A. F. Subar, T. Mouw, P. Hartge, L. M. Morton, R. Stolzenberg-Solomon, et al., "Consumption of Aspartame-Containing Beverages and Incidence of Hematopoietic and Brain Malignancies," *Cancer Epidemiology, Biomarkers & Prevention* 15, no. 9 (2006): 1654–59.

145   *scientists claimed that aspartame given to rats:* M. Soffritti, F. Belpoggi, D. Degli Esposti, and L. Lambertini, "Aspartame Induces Lymphomas and Leukaemias in Rats," *European Journal of Oncology* 10, no. 2 (2005): 107–16.

a 1998 randomized controlled trial: P. A. Spiers, L. Sabounjian, A. Reiner, D. K. Myers, J. Wurtman, and D. L. Schomer, "Aspartame: Neuropsychologic and Neurophysiologic Evaluation of Acute and Chronic Effects," *American Journal of Clinical Nutrition* 68, no. 3 (1998): 531–37.

146   *another randomized controlled trial, in 1994:* B. A. Shaywitz, C. M. Sullivan, G. M. Anderson, S. M. Gillespie, B. Sullivan, and S. E. Shaywitz, "Aspartame, Behavior, and Cognitive Function in Children with Attention Deficit Disorder," *Pediatrics* 93, no. 1 (1994): 70–75.

A safety review: B. A. Magnuson, G. A. Burdock, J. Doull, R. M. Kroes, G. M. Marsh, M. W. Pariza, et al., "Aspartame: A Safety Evaluation Based on Current Use Levels, Regulations, and Toxicological and Epidemiological Studies," *Critical Reviews in Toxicology* 37, no. 8 (2007): 629–727.

a huge study published in Nature: J. Suez, T. Korem, D. Zeevi, G. Zilberman-Schapira, C. A. Thaiss, O. Maza, et al., "Artificial Sweeteners Induce Glucose Intolerance by Altering the Gut Microbiota," *Nature* 514, no. 7521 (2014): 181–86.

148   *study published in the journal* Obesity: S. P. Fowler, K. Williams, R. G. Resendez, K. J. Hunt, H. P. Hazuda, and M. P. Stern, "Fueling the Obesity Epidemic? Artificially Sweetened Beverage Use and Long-Term Weight Gain," *Obesity* 16, no. 8 (2008): 1894–1900.

another study cropped up: C. W. Chia, M. Shardell, T. Tanaka, D. D. Liu, K. S. Gravenstein, E. M. Simonsick, et al., "Chronic Low-Calorie Sweetener Use and Risk of Abdominal Obesity Among Older Adults: A Cohort Study," *PLOS ONE* 11, no. 11 (2016): e0167241.

149   *known as* reverse causality: M. A. Pereira, "Diet Beverages and the Risk of Obesity, Dia-
      betes, and Cardiovascular Disease: A Review of the Evidence," *Nutrition Reviews* 71, no.
      7 (2013): 433–40.

150   *researchers published the results of a trial:* D. F. Tate, G. Turner-McGrievy, E. Lyons, J.
      Stevens, K. Erickson, K. Polzien, et al., "Replacing Caloric Beverages with Water or Diet
      Beverages for Weight Loss in Adults: Main Results of the Choose Healthy Options Con-
      sciously Everyday (CHOICE) Randomized Clinical Trial," *American Journal of Clinical
      Nutrition* 95, no. 3 (2012): 555–63.

      published in the American Journal of Clinical Nutrition: P. E. Miller and V. Perez, "Low-
      Calorie Sweeteners and Body Weight and Composition: A Meta-analysis of Random-
      ized Controlled Trials and Prospective Cohort Studies," *American Journal of Clinical
      Nutrition* 100, no. 3 (2014): 765–77.

151   *artificial sweetener fans:* P. Rosenthal, "Fading Diet Pepsi Brings Back Sweetener That
      Sickens Rats but Tastes Better," *Chicago Tribune,* June 28, 2016, http://www.chicagotri
      bune.com/business/ct-rosenthal-diet-pepsi-aspartame-rats-0628-biz-20160627-col
      umn.html.

10. MSG

156   *published in the prestigious medical journal:* A. J. Wakefield, S. H. Murch, A. Anthony, J.
      Linnell, D. M. Casson, M. Malik, et al., "RETRACTED: Ileal-Lymphoid-Nodular Hyper-
      plasia, Non-specific Colitis, and Pervasive Developmental Disorder in Children," *Lan-
      cet* 351, no. 9103 (1998): 637–41.

      later investigation found: B. Deer, "How the Case Against the MMR Vaccine Was Fixed,"
      BMJ 342 (2011): c5347.

157   *try to set the record straight:* A. E. Carroll, "JAMA Forum: When Good Science Doesn't
      Sway Minds, It's Time to Move On," *@newsatJAMA* (blog), *JAMA,* May 6, 2015, https://
      newsatjama.jama.com/2015/05/06/jama-forum-when-good-science-doesnt-sway-
      minds-its-time-to-move-on/.

158   *I wouldn't advocate:* L. C. Dolan, R. A. Matulka, and G. A. Burdock, "Naturally Occur-
      ring Food Toxins," *Toxins* 2, no. 9 (2010): 2289–2332.

      additive carrageenan in their products: Food Babe, "Watch Out for This Carcinogen in
      Your Organic Food," last updated February 24, 2015, http://foodbabe.com/2012/05/22/
      watch-out-for-this-carcinogen-in-your-organic-food.

      provided a link to a report: Food Babe, "BREAKING: Major Company Removing Con-
      troversial Ingredient Carrageenan Because Of You!," August 19, 2014, http://foodbabe.
      com/2014/08/19/breaking-major-company-removing-controversial-ingredient-carra
      geenan-because-of-you.

159   *the WHO has labeled:* "List of Classifications," World Health Organization, Interna-
      tional Agency for Research on Cancer, http://monographs.iarc.fr/ENG/Classifica
      tion/.

      directed their wrath at Subway: Food Babe, "The One Thing Subway Is Still Hiding from
      All of Us!," February 7, 2014, http://foodbabe.com/2014/02/07/subway-update/.

      basically eating yoga mats: Food Babe, "Subway: Stop Using Dangerous Chemicals In
      Your Bread," n.d., http://foodbabe.com/subway/.

164   *"Chinese-Restaurant Syndrome":* Robert Ho Man Kwok, "Chinese-Restaurant Syndrome," letter, *New England Journal of Medicine* 278, no. 14 (1968): 796.

       the New York Times *joined the fray:* R. D. Lyons, "Chinese Restaurant Syndrome Puzzles Doctors," *New York Times,* May 19, 1968, 68.

       articles sought to question those beliefs: I. Mosby, "'That Won-Ton Soup Headache': The Chinese Restaurant Syndrome, MSG and the Making of American Food, 1968–1980," *Social History of Medicine* 22, no. 1 (2009): 133–51.

165   *"That Won-Ton Soup Headache":* P. L. Raymer, "That Won-Ton Soup Headache," *New York Times,* April 20, 1977, http://www.nytimes.com/1977/04/20/archives/westchester-weekly-that-wonton-soup-headache.html.

       somewhat based in racism: Mosby, "'That Won-Ton Soup Headache.'"

       study published in Science: J. W. Olney, "Brain Lesions, Obesity, and Other Disturbances in Mice Treated with Monosodium Glutamate," *Science* 164, no. 3880 (1969): 719.

       researchers were feeding 20 grams of MSG: H. Ohguro, H. Katsushima, I. Maruyama, T. Maeda, S. Yanagihashi, T. Metoki, et al., "A High Dietary Intake of Sodium Glutamate as Flavoring (Ajinomoto) Causes Gross Changes in Retinal Morphology and Function," *Experimental Eye Research* 75, no. 3 (2002): 307–15.

       the average amount: "Questions and Answers on Monosodium Glutamate (MSG)," U.S. Food and Drug Administration, November 19, 2012, https://www.fda.gov/Food/IngredientsPackagingLabeling/FoodAdditivesIngredients/ucm328728.htm.

       the famous star of TV's Bonanza: Mosby, "'That Won-Ton Soup Headache.'"

       more than baby formula and cow's milk: C. Agostoni, B. Carratù, C. Boniglia, A. M. Lammardo, E. Riva, and E. Sanzini, "Free Glutamine and Glutamic Acid Increase in Human Milk Through a Three-Month Lactation Period," *Journal of Pediatric Gastroenterology and Nutrition* 31, no. 5 (2000): 508–12.

166   *high levels of histamine:* K. W. Chin, M. M. Garriga, and D. D. Metcalfe, "The Histamine Content of Oriental Foods," *Food and Chemical Toxicology* 27, no. 5 (1989): 283–87.

167   *a 1993 study published in the journal:* L. Tarasoff and M. F. Kelly, "Monosodium L-glutamate: A Double-Blind Study and Review," *Food and Chemical Toxicology* 31, no. 12 (1993): 1019–35.

168   *no MSG-induced asthma effects:* R. K. Woods, J. M. Weiner, F. Thien, M. Abramson, and E. H. Walters, "The Effects of Monosodium Glutamate in Adults with Asthma Who Perceive Themselves to Be Monosodium Glutamate-Intolerant," *Journal of Allergy and Clinical Immunology,* pt. 1, 101, no. 6 (1998): 762–71.

       a randomized controlled trial of one hundred people: K. M. Woessner, R. A. Simon, and D. D. Stevenson, "Monosodium Glutamate Sensitivity in Asthma," *Journal of Allergy and Clinical Immunology,* pt. 1, 104, no. 2 (1999): 305–10.

       researchers published a study so thorough: R. S. Geha, A. Beise, C. Ren, R. Patterson, P. A. Greenberger, L. C. Grammer, et al., "Multicenter, Double-Blind, Placebo-Controlled, Multiple-Challenge Evaluation of Reported Reactions to Monosodium Glutamate," *Journal of Allergy and Clinical Immunology* 106, no. 5 (2000): 973–80.

11. NON-ORGANIC FOODS

173   *went to the USDA website:* National Organic Program, "Organic Production and Handling Standards" (U.S. Department of Agriculture, October 2002; updated October 2011), https://www.ams.usda.gov/sites/default/files/media/Organic%20Production-Handling%20Standards.pdf.

175   *data on the price differences:* A. Carlson, "Investigating Retail Price Premiums for Organic Foods," *Amber Waves,* May 24, 2016, https://www.ers.usda.gov/amber-waves/2016/may/investigating-retail-price-premiums-for-organic-foods/.
       about 5% of the spinach: Ibid.

176   *most thorough study I've seen:* C. Smith-Spangler, M. L. Brandeau, G. E. Hunter, J. C. Bavinger, M. Pearson, P. J. Eschbach, et al., "Are Organic Foods Safer or Healthier Than Conventional Alternatives? A Systematic Review," *Annals of Internal Medicine* 157, no. 5 (2012): 348–66.

179   *a newer study in the* British Journal of Nutrition: M. Baranski, D. Srednicka-Tober, N. Volakakis, C. Seal, R. Sanderson, G. B. Stewart, et al., "Higher Antioxidant and Lower Cadmium Concentrations and Lower Incidence of Pesticide Residues in Organically Grown Crops: A Systematic Literature Review and Meta-analyses," *British Journal of Nutrition* 112, no. 5 (2014): 794–811.
       "most extensive analysis" of its kind: Newcastle University, "Organic vs Non-organic Food," press release, October 8, 2015, http://www.ncl.ac.uk/press/news/2015/10/organicvsnon-organicfood/.

180   *Antioxidants are chemical compounds:* "Antioxidants," MedlinePlus, National Library of Medicine, last updated May 5, 2017, https://medlineplus.gov/antioxidants.html.
       Various studies on vitamin E: I. M. Lee, N. R. Cook, J. M. Gaziano, D. Gordon, P. M. Ridker, J. E. Manson, et al., "Vitamin E in the Primary Prevention of Cardiovascular Disease and Cancer: The Women's Health Study; A Randomized Controlled Trial," *JAMA* 294, no. 1 (2005): 56–65; The HOPE and HOPE-TOO Trial Investigators, "Effects of Long-Term Vitamin E Supplementation on Cardiovascular Events and Cancer: A Randomized Controlled Trial," *JAMA* 293, no. 11 (2005): 1338–47; GISSI-Prevenzione Investigators, "Dietary Supplementation with n-3 Polyunsaturated Fatty Acids and Vitamin E After Myocardial Infarction: Results of the GISSI-Prevenzione Trial," *Lancet* 354, no. 9177 (1999): 447–55.
       Other studies focusing on beta-carotene: C. H. Hennekens, J. E. Buring, J. E. Manson, M. Stampfer, B. Rosner, N. R. Cook, et al., "Lack of Effect of Long-Term Supplementation with Beta Carotene on the Incidence of Malignant Neoplasms and Cardiovascular Disease," *New England Journal of Medicine* 334, no. 18 (1996): 1145–49.
       more studies looking at mixtures of antioxidants: N. R. Cook, C. M. Albert, J. M. Gaziano, E. Zaharris, J. MacFadyen, E. Danielson, et al., "A Randomized Factorial Trial of Vitamins C and E and Beta Carotene in the Secondary Prevention of Cardiovascular Events in Women: Results from the Women's Antioxidant Cardiovascular Study," *Archives of Internal Medicine* 167, no. 15 (2007): 1610–18; S. Hercberg, P. Galan, P. Preziosi, S. Bertrais, L. Mennen, D. Malvy, et al. "The SU.VI.MAX Study: A Randomized, Placebo-Controlled Trial of the Health Effects of Antioxidant Vitamins and Minerals," *Archives of Internal Medicine* 164, no. 21 (2004): 2335–42.

182   *one of the best summaries I've read:* T. Haspel, "Is Organic Agriculture Really Better for the Environment?," *Washington Post,* May 14, 2016.

183   *the government's standards:* C. Wilcox, "Mythbusting 101: Organic Farming > Conventional Agriculture," *Science Sushi* (blog), *Scientific American,* July 18, 2011, https://blogs.scientificamerican.com/science-sushi/httpblogsscientificamericancomscience-sushi20110718mythbusting-101-organic-farming-conventional-agriculture/.

       limits on the amount of rotenone: P. Caboni, T. B. Sherer, N. Zhang, G. Taylor, H. M. Na, J. T. Greenamyre, et al., "Rotenone, Deguelin, Their Metabolites, and the Rat Model of Parkinson's Disease," *Chemical Research in Toxicology* 17, no. 11, (2004): 1540–48.

185   *only about 4% of all food that's sold:* "Organic Market Overview," U.S. Department of Agriculture, Economic Research Service, last updated April 4, 2017, https://www.ers.usda.gov/topics/natural-resources-environment/organic-agriculture/organic-market-overview/.

       In many countries in Europe: K. Heinze, "European Organic Market Grew to More Than 26 Billion Euros in 2014," *Organic-market.info,* February 23, 2016, http://organic-market.info/news-in-brief-and-reports-article/european-organic-market-grew-to-more-than-26-billion-euros-in-2014.html.

CONCLUSION

192   *throw research at me that says so:* S. Bowen, S. Elliott, and J. Brenton, "The Joy of Cooking?," *Contexts* 13, no. 3 (2014): 20–25.

195   *benefits beyond nutrition:* A. E. Carroll, "Obesity Interventions Can Improve More Than Just Body Mass Index," *JAMA Pediatrics* 167, no. 11 (2013): 1002–3.

INDEX